The Miracle Tree

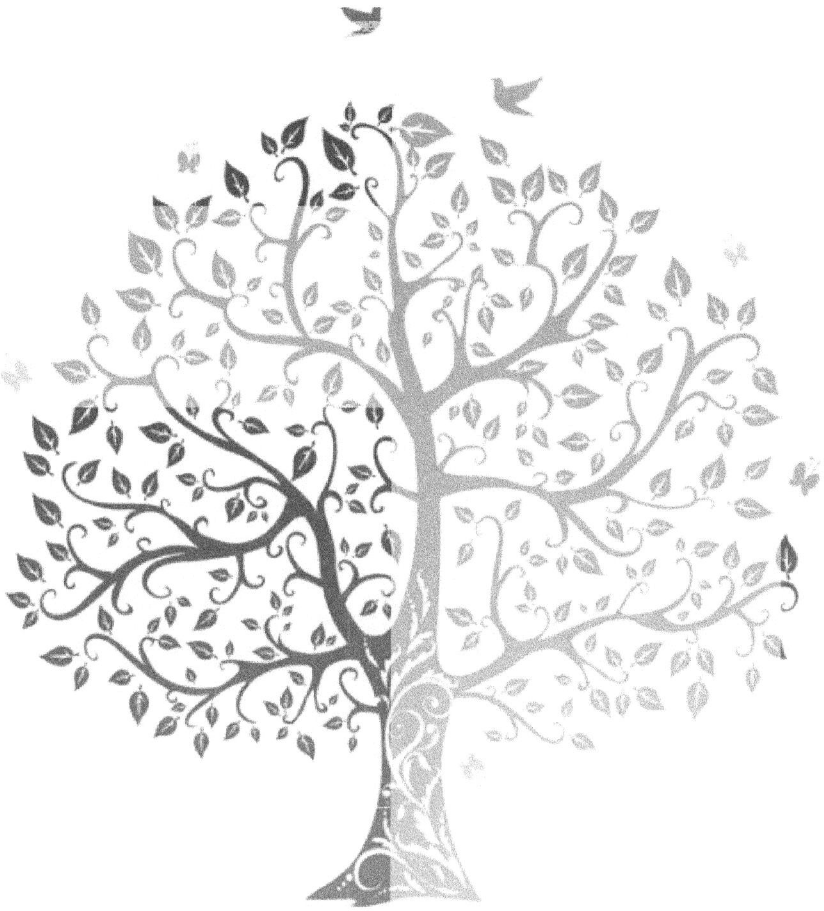

by Doug Mollo

Book Published and Edited

by *Do Life Big Network*

www.dolifebigger.com/book

THE MIRACLE TREE

MORINGA

Doug Mollo Owner

Creator Of Moringa Health

FORWARD: WHO I AM

MISSIONARY, HEALER, VISIONARY

ENTREPRENEUR, FORMULATOR

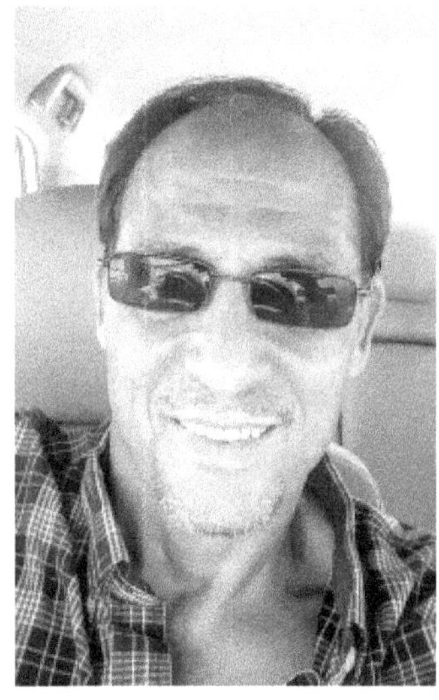

Hi Im, Doug often referred to as
Dougie Moringa Mollo.

Welcome to a grand adventure that stems the duration of many
decades, of countless hours, days and weeks of life.

My true story begins when I found myself lying on my back on South Beach in Florida looking up from the sandy shores of Miami's playa de sol. I had just performed an acrobatic marvel where I failed to rotate a back aerial somersault and came **straight down on my head**. God did not create our vertebrae in such a way as to absorb such an impact that I delivered to my neck. As I lay on the beach staring into the blue sky spotted with puffy white cumulous clouds I instantly knew exactly what I had done. After years of coaching top Florida state champion gymnastic teams, and diving countless times to save little necks from breaking, my fate was clear. Lying there with my head on a soft sandy patch my body was floating six inches off the ground and had no feeling whatsoever. As I looked to the clouds I began a series of self-talk that would change my life forever.

You see I was never much of a spiritual guy. Oh I went to church for years with my parents and living across the street from St Ann's, the shadow of the cross ever loomed over my life as a clear acknowledgment of a higher power. I went through life carrying a deep-rooted belief that God existed. I always knew he was there around me and protecting me like protective bubble wrap, always waiting to pick me up and bail me out. This day lying on the beach was very different as it was the very first time I actually turned and **looked into his face**. As I lie there on sunny south beach the entire world faded away, and I looked to the sky and said, "Lord take this cup from me". Being a twenty-five season gymnastic coach you see I knew exactly what I had done. Countless times I have stretched my hands out to save a young girl from such a fate as this. As I lie on the beach I know that I was paralyzed. I had come straight down on my neck and I had fully compressed my 4-5 / 5-6 vertebrae in such a way that I had severed my spinal column. Later I found out that I went as far as I possibly could have without a full separation, and by the grace of God there was a very small fraction that was still intact. One more **hair sized split** and I could have been called Christopher Reave the

My Backflip On a Beach

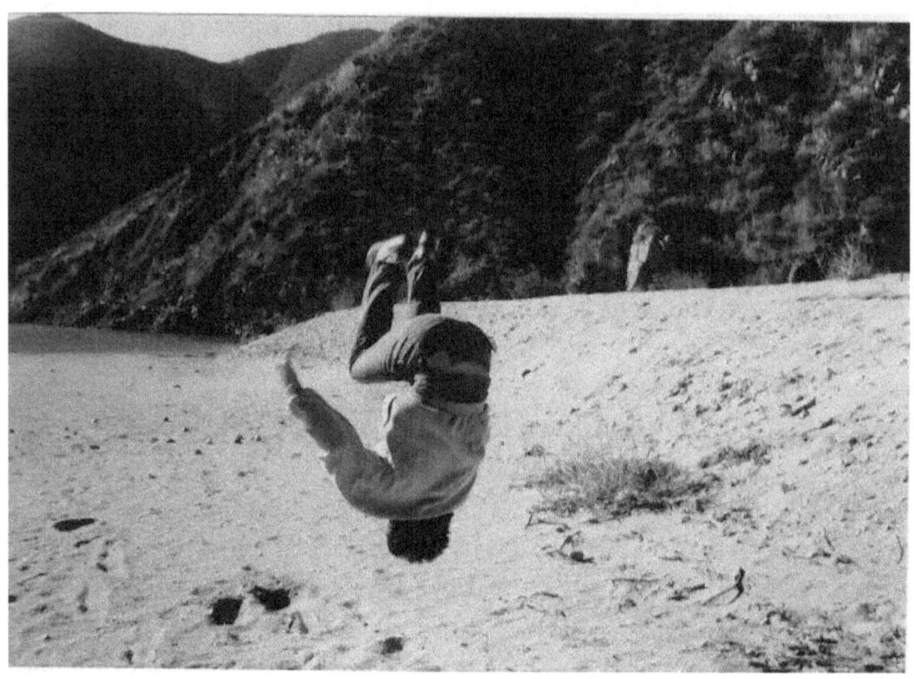

second. God knew I was no "super man", just a reckless show off trying to trying to impress my date. As I stared into the Miami sky, I began to speak with God. Though extremely clichéd, I actually did uses Jesus's own words. "take this cup from me".

I knew right there on the spot that my life as I knew it was going to change **forever.** God physically appeared to me as the typical aged bearded spirit of wisdom, and as I looked upon his loving face he spoke these words to me, "deal with it". You see at the time he knew that tough love were the only words I understood. Right there at that time I began to accept that this was the way I would be, that my life as I knew it would all be at an end. All the years of saving others from such a fate would come back to me in buckets of irony. As I lie there floating I had a peace beyond all comprehension, you see as I said before I had always known God existed but I had never **looked Him in the face** before. Now as I lie there I finally looked into the eyes of God himself, all the while coming to terms with my new reality. Life in a <u>wheelchair</u> was a stark reality to swallow for someone who was so full of life.

The natural progression of things when a serious accident occurs is a state of trauma and shock. The body goes into a protective state. Some survivors of severe injury can lose organ function, generally starting with the lungs and kidneys and then moving to the liver and intestines. This potentially deadly condition, called multiple organ dysfunction syndrome (MODS), can happen early if people go into shock, when their tissues don't receive adequate oxygen. It can also occur later in the recovery process. It's not just organs that can behave differently after trauma; genes can, too.

A nationwide team headed by Tompkins conducted a 10-year study of hospital patients whose conditions included **severe blunt trauma**. The researchers determined that all the blunt trauma cases requiring intensive care incited a "genomic storm" in which 80 percent of the genes controlling immune activity behaved differently in the first 4 weeks following the injury than they did in a healthy individual. Another potential result of trauma is body-wide inflammation, or sepsis. Following a traumatic injury, the body produces a flood of white blood cells that can secrete a protein called HMGB1. This protein contributes to septic inflammation, which can be life threatening. No matter how many books or internet sites you research and study, there are no cases that state someone does not go into shock of some type, and just as rare are cases of people mentally coming to grips with the new state of affaires.

The Miami paramedics arrived on the scene, and after assessing my situation re-routed me to Jackson memorial hospital, one of the best hospitals for trauma in the country. The long and the short of it is that I was given a 30% percent chance of walking again, and after a 7 hour emergency operation and being spared from temple mounted screw in halo, after six months of quality care, God saw it to allow me to walk again. I still visit Jackson "pancake ward" where I was destine to be flipped like a pancake as less fortunate quadriplegics are to this very day. Still when I visit the nurses and I cry and I have been lovingly nick named the "Miracle Man".

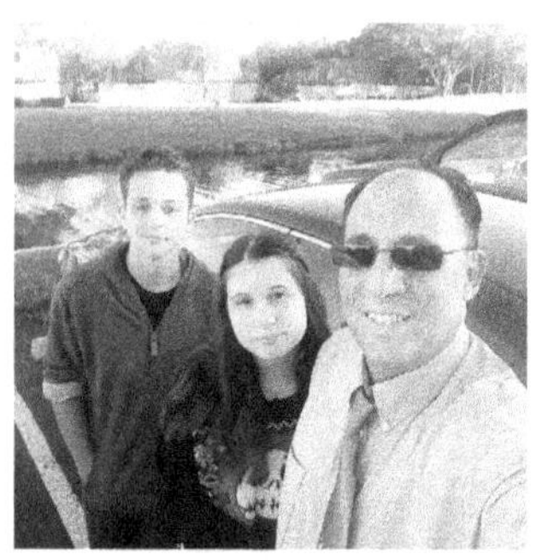

So why do I tell you all of this in a book that is named the Miracle Tree? Well I tell you because God had taken me through a wild training seminar called **life**. Please allow me to embellish where God has brought me, and keep in mind I do not tell you this to impress but to impress upon you Gods leading, and omnipotent hand in our life. I have had opportunity to run a cosmeceutical formulation, and distribution company as well as digital technology company provider of computer networking and digital surveillance. For a span of twenty-four years I gained experience in marketing, and sales. My prominent focus has been global distribution of health and wellness products both traditionally and through e-commerce and interactive mediums. I have had the pleasure to both work, and learn from the best in the business. I have developed a passion to help others reach and obtain their dreams. God has helped me grow a strong traditional business foundation, and first hand web site production experience, as a partner in an Internet advertising agency. He has positioned me for such a time as this. As a full time gymnastic coach, and amateur clinical nutritionist, I have a heart for kids and health. He has dedicated my heart to self-improvement and spiritual growth for others and myself.

As I started 2017, I found myself lacking direction and unemployed. I was open to God's direction and I always knew that I was spared from a like in a wheelchair for a reason. My heart to help others and a desire to mix my faith with holistic health has brought me to a new place of hope as I follow His lead as I climb the Tree of Life.

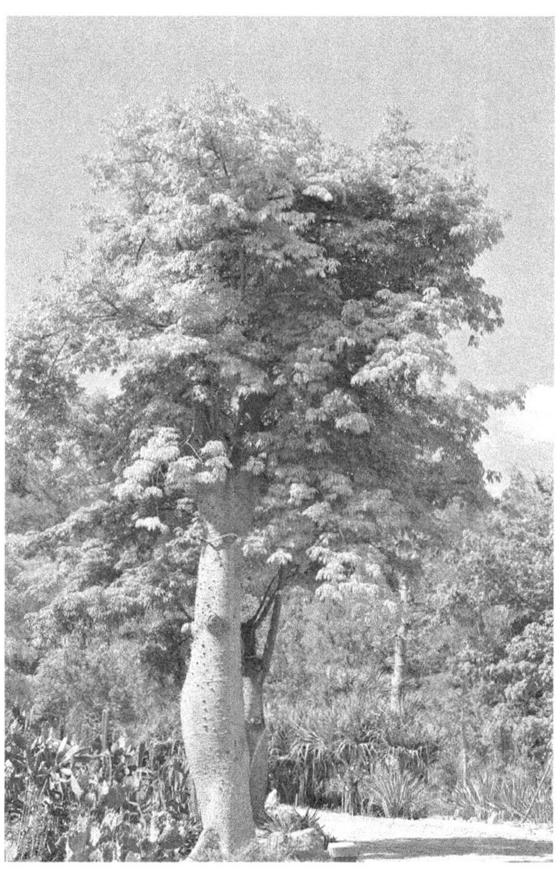

HOW I FOUND THE TREE

DIVINE INTERVENTION

Divine Intervention is a special phrase for me as for many years I was seeking Gods' will in my life and for a series of four or five years a self funded a ministry called Di Mission Web. A web design company that developed websites for Christian ministries worldwide. Di stood for Divine Intervention.

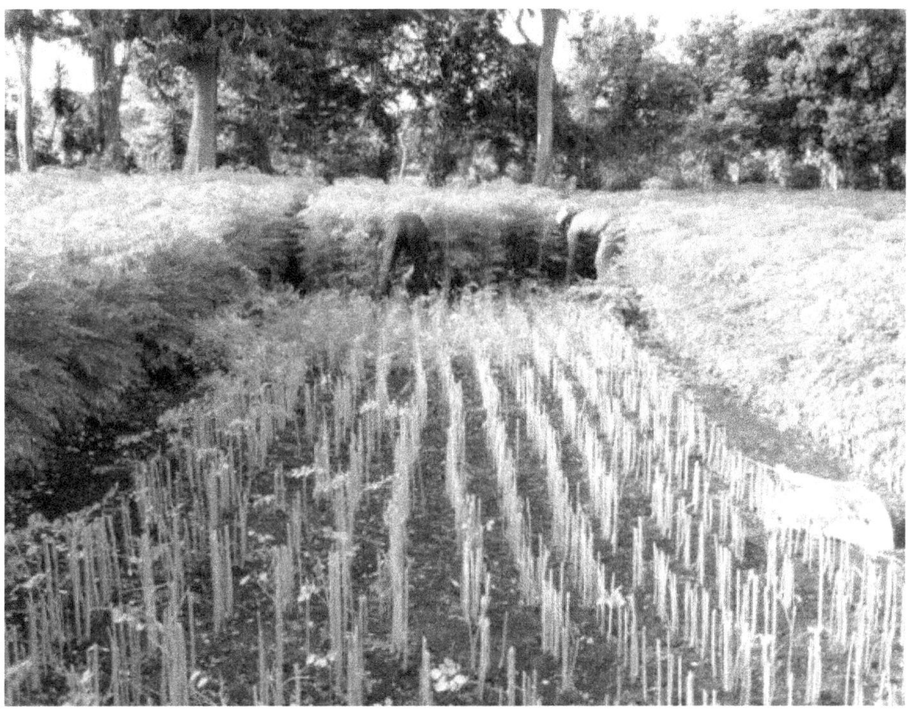

On a mild winter night in south Florida I received and email from a sister in Christ named Mary. Mary sent me a video of a Latin botanist who was searching for healing herbs. At first I almost didn't watch the video because I thought it was just another intro promo for an MLM company. Though I am not against MLM, I was not seeking out that type of business model. As a matter of fact I was not seeking anything at the time other than a stronger relationship with God. I decided to continue to watch the video as the announcer began to explain how this man found a tree whose leaves have incredible healing properties. He was not the first to find this tree, but it was new to him, as it was new to me. The more I watched the more my spirit was stirred and the more intrigued I became. I ended up not leaving my computer for about three full days. I became obsessed with what I was learning about this mysterious tree. The more I researched the more interested I became.

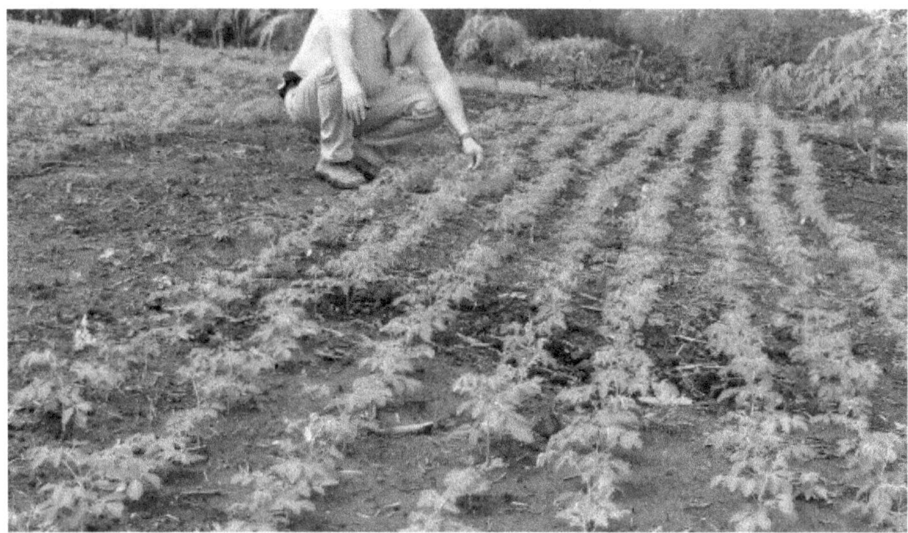

After several weeks of research I had found out that over 80% of the word population knew about the medicinal benefits of the Miracle Tree and only 6% of the USA population had even heard of it. Around the world the tree had many different names here are just a few:

GLOBAL MORINGA TREE NAMES

ENGLISH: Horseradish tree, Radish tree, Drumstick tree, Mother's Best Friend, West Indian ben.

FRENCH: Bèn ailé, Benzolive.

AFRICA: BURKINA FASO: Argentiga, Arzam tigha ("The tree of paradise"). (Fulfuldé): Guilgandani, Gigandjah.

GHANA: (Ewe): Yevu-ti.

KENYA: (Swahili): Mlonge, Mronge, Mrongo, Mlongo, Mzunze, Mzungu.

MALAWI: (Chichewa): Cham'mwanba, Kangaluni. (Yao): Kalokola. (Senna): Nsangoa.

NIGER: (Hausa): Zôgala gandi. (Zarma): Windi-bundu. NIGERIA: (Fulani): Gawara, Konamarade, Rini maka, Habiwal hausa. (Hausa): Zogall, Zogalla-gandi, Bagaruwar maka,Bagaruwar masar, Shipka hali, Shuka halinka, Barambo, Koraukin zaila, Rimin turawa, Rimin nacara. (Ibo): Ikwe oyibo. (Yoruba): Ewe ile, Ewe igbale, Idagbo monoye ("The tree which grows crazily").

SENEGAL: (Wolof): Neverday, Nébéday. (Serer): Nébéday. SUDAN: (Arabic): Ruwag, Alim, Halim, Shagara al ruwag. TOGO: (Dagomba): Baganlua, Bagaelean.

ZIMBABWE: (Tonga): Mupulanga, Zakalanda. BURMA: Dandalonbin.

CAMBODIA: Ben ailé, Daem mrum. INDIA: (Bengalese): Sajna. (Gujarati): Suragavo. (Hindi): Shajmah, Shajna, Segra. (Malayam): Sigru, Moringa, Muringa. (Marathi): Sujna, Shevga. (Oriya): Munigha, Sajina. (Punjabese): Sanjina, Soanjana. (Sanskrit): Sobhan jana. (Tamil): Murungai. (Telegu): Sajana.

INDONESIA: Kalor, Kelor.

PHILIPPINES: Mulangai, Mulangay.

COLOMBIA: Angela.

COSTA RICA: Marango.

DOMINICAN REPUBLIC: Palo de aceiti, Palo de abejas, Libertad.

EL SALVADOR: Teberinto.

GUADALOUPE: Moloko, Ben-ailé.

GUATAMALA: Perlas, Paraiso blanco.

GUIANA: Saijhan. HAITI: Benzolive, Benzolivier, Ben oleifere, Bambou-bananier, Graines benne.

HONDURAS: Maranga calalu.

PANAMA: Jacinto.

PUERTO RICO: Resada, Ben, Jasmin francés.

SURINAM Kelor, Peperwortel boom. ALSO: Acacia, Aceite, Arbol de las perlas, Arbol do los aspáragos, Bamboubamamoer, Benbom, Benboom, Brenoili, Cedro, Cenauro, Chinto borrego, Chuva de prata, Desengaño, Gailito, Goma, Guaireña, Hoja de sen, Jacinto, Macasar, Maloko, Malungay, Marenque, Moongay, Moriengo, Moringa, Naragno, Noz de bem, Orenga, Orselli, Palo de geringa, Palo jeringa, Paraiso, Paraiso de españa, Paraiso extranjero, Paraiso francés, Perlas del oriente, Pois quinique, Quiabo de tres quinas, Sainto John, Salaster, Salibau, Sen, Seringa.

As a businessperson I was extremely excited about the prospect of exposing this lost treasure to the US population, as someone who was interested in holistic healing, and helping others I was enthusiastic about the prospects of its use. I began to develop international contacts seeking to import for distribution. I contacted distributors in India, Philippians, Brazil and others. However, no matter how many government, medical, organic documents I received validating the high quality and organic integrity of the product I received, physical inspection would fall short. You see I was seeking a quality for myself, and my family that I would be comfortable with to use and to offer to others.

However, every time I received product it would fall short of my expectations. Green product would arrive brown. Processed powder would be gritty, and analysis would expose impurities. Temperature fluctuations in transport, required radiation from customs and poor processing procedures would further degrade the nutritional integrity of the product.

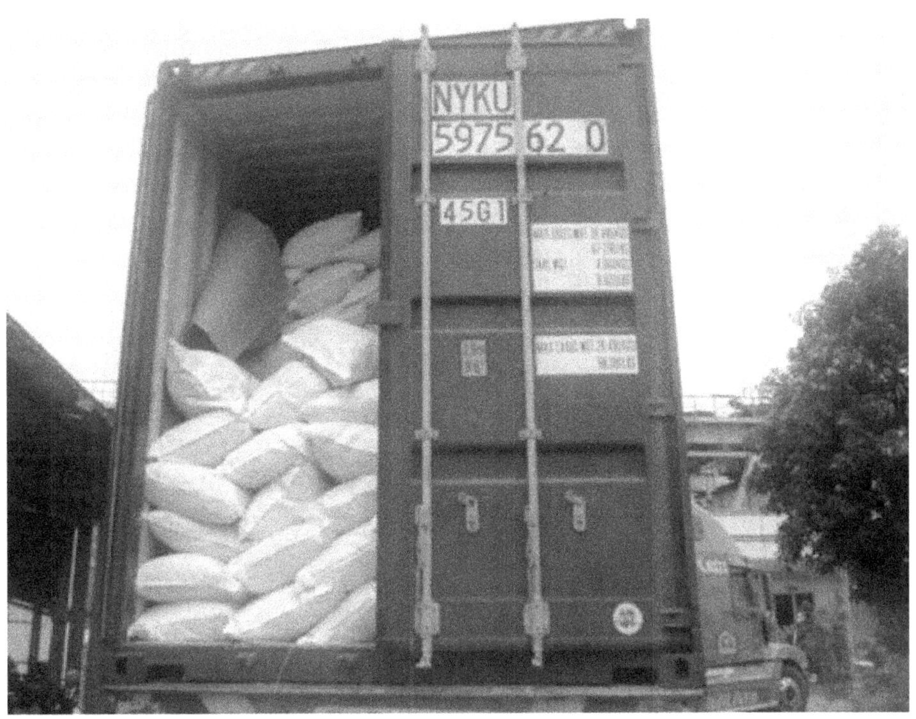

I became more and more frustrated and as I began to germinate my own seeds for personal use felt less confident that I would ever be able to provide a top quality product to the US general public, and then it happened. Miracously, I found a USA based grower in California who was willing to provide me product for distribution.

After receiving his product and further review it became clear to me that this company was simply buying most of their product over seas. Though they had good intentions the market would just not make it cost affective for them to solely base production on US soil. The market was forcing them to compromise. I however, had no tolerance for this kind of compromise and was determined to provide USA grown Moringa to the world market.

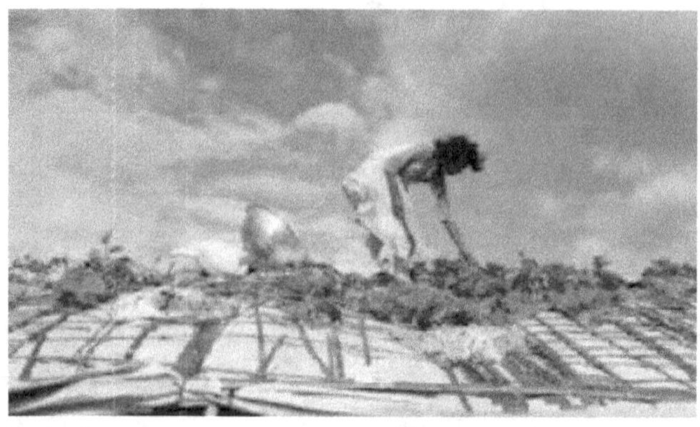

Not long after this final setback **God intervened**, and I stumbled on to a local Florida manufacturer how was to prove a most valuable asset to my business model.

For discussion purposes lets just call this person Steve. Well Steve was a God sent and defiantly a "Di", Divine Intervention. You see Steve had a very interesting story. For many years Steve served as a Green Barrett for the Argentinian army. Until one day where he was dropped off in the Amazon jungle. He was left for dead, and ended up spending five years with the Amazonian natives and became a student of the tribal healers.

True Shamans and the original herbalists, worked side by side to take Steve in as family, and to teach him the arts of healing using rain forest herbs, and hidden tribal secrets. Many years later Steve settled in Florida and began to cultivate and cross bread Moringa Oliefera plants. He created, and develops the finest strain of Moringa in the world. Not unlike the cannabis cultivators Steve cross bread plant stems and seeds always testing and re-testing. Through trial-and-error, he ended up developing the finest Moringa available on planet earth, grown right here in the good old USA. By an act of God I stumbled on the finest high quality product available today right in my own backyard. You see this story is quite incredible but it does not stop there. If you recall I was not looking for a business, and I was most certainly not looking for a botanical business. God had a plan he planted a seed, and He was just getting started.

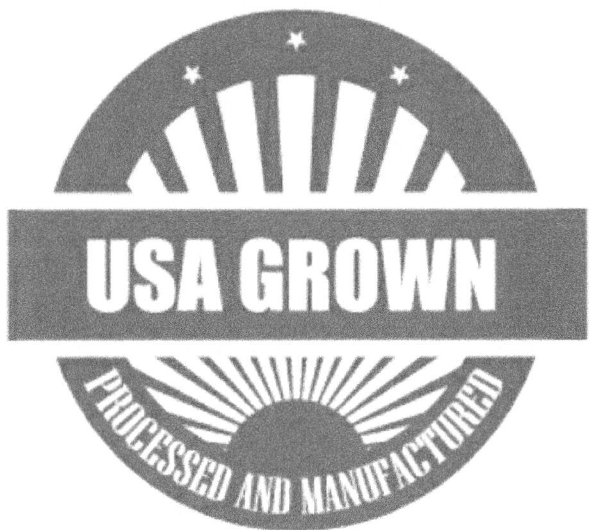

It turned out that Steve was not only developing the best Moringa in the world but for years he had been developing, and testing Moringa based rain forest blend formulations. These formulations had the potential to aid in the curing a broad spectrum of illnesses and diseases. Of course as a botanical supplement company, I was not able to make claims that I had the solution to get diabetics off their medication in two weeks, nor could I promise to remove ADAD sufferers from the use of Adderall, or help to lower blood pressure in heart disease patients but the truth was we could. We will visit more of these herbal formulations in chapter 4.

The bottom line was that God had a plan and he was using me to deliver health and wellness to the masses.

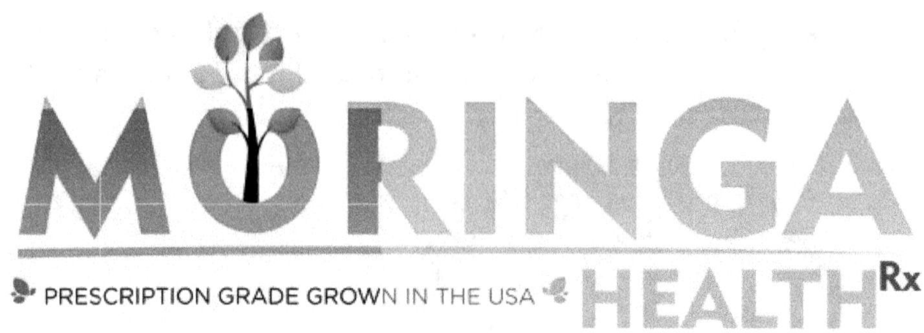

Moringa Health was born.

Chapter:2

QUALITY CONTROL

IMPORTS AND CORPORATE PROFITS

I am a person who likes to find the **best** in people, and conversely I like to think the best of companies as well. The division of corporations states that a company is to be treated as and individual, and those companies are run by individuals, and are to be honest and forth right in all of their practices. Generally, I think that most companies start out with the best intentions and want to do good in the world, and do well by their customers. However, somewhere along the line they get sidetracked. After all happy customers make loyal purchasers, and loyalty is good for business. So than what happens? Why are so many companies just not doing the right thing? One word, **<u>greed</u>**.

Without being cynical or too harsh, it is really a combination of greed, and practicality. Companies, simply have to be competitive. With so many companies vying for the same piece of the market share, a funnel is created that sucks companies down to the lowest level of compromise.

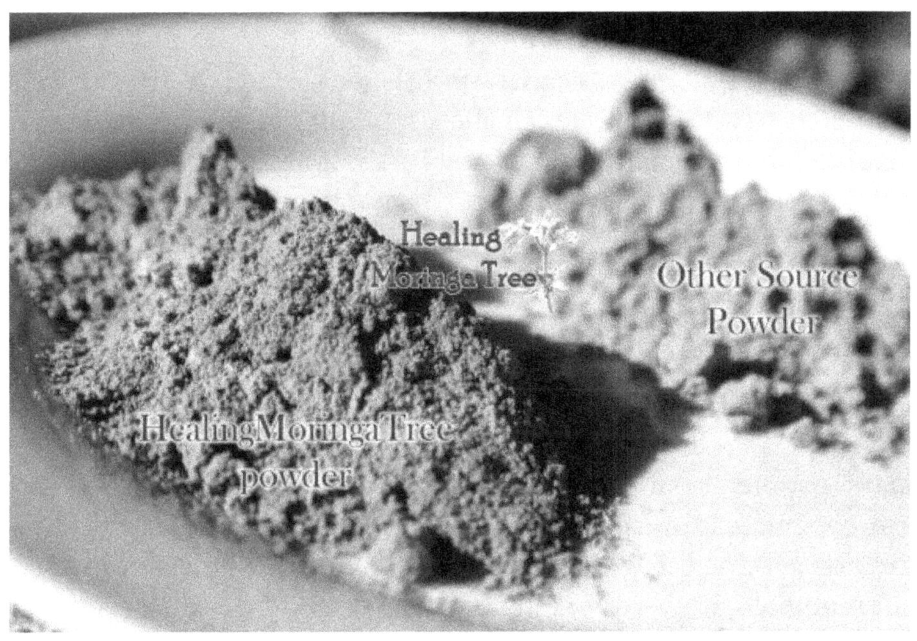

We all have to live by some level of a moral compass. Something has to guide our decisions and direct our steps. Unfortunately, one bad step after another tends to create a path in the wrong direction. The stairs seem to lead downward, and climbing back up is virtually impossible. So many companies set out to do the right thing,   to be the standard in their given industry, and eventually by making small steady compromises fall deeper into market despair. The bottom line becomes the only thing of importance, and the competitive edge is governed by profitability, leaving integrity as a thin margin.

The supplement world is perhaps no better or worse than any other market, in that compromise is at the forefront of the barrel race. One company rolling over another to market and coerce their prospective client into believing theirs is better then the next. Companies often have no choice but to follow the leader to the cheapest pathway to success in production, often leading to manipulative marketing and deceiving sales tactics.

The New York Times recently published an article that stated that 60% of all companies in the supplement industry had misleading labels in that most of the ingredients on the label were not in the product. It went on to say that most did not even have the main ingredient on the front of the label in the product at all. Dr Gupta and recognized news authority in the medical community recently sighted a study stating that most CBD companies did not have the proper (mg) listed on the label that was actually in the product.

Many people are not getting what they pay for. They are lead to believe misleading marketing and sales pitches. Ultimately they are not getting tat which they are paying for, when it comes to supplements, herbs, oils, and botanicals.

Moringa companies are no different, and it is one of the main reasons I am writing this book. It is said that if you write a book you are immediately perceived as being an expert in that given field. That may or may not be so, however I do know that it is important for people to know the truth. Jesus said, it you know the truth the truth will set you free. No doubt on a spiritual level Jesus is the truth and the life, and there is no other way to the Father then through the Son. I also believe that sheading he light on the Moringa tree can, and will set some people free. It has become my mission in life to educate people about the truth both spiritually, and physically.

It is most important to me that you understand not only the importance of Moringa Oliefera as an incredible super food, and preventative health care option, but I want you to come away knowing that not all Moringa products are the same. As the owner and founder of Moringa Health it is important to me that you know the truth. Before you run out there, and you buy something because it says it contains Moringa think again. Just because it contains Moringa does not necessarily mean that it is nutritionally good for you.

Moringa Health brings you the finest Moringa grown on the planet, and it is grown right here locally in the USA. Through years of painstaking formulation of the finest rain forest ingredients, Moringa Health is confident and proud to being you nothing but the best. When you buy Moringa Health you know your getting superior grade Moringa Grown In The USA with no fillers, impurities or compromises.

Moringa Health is the worlds standard for high grade sourced Moringa Oleifera, and Moringa based products. Basically, when an organic super-food exhibits a bright green color, crisper fullness of flavor and density, it is indicating higher concentrations of nutrients, quality and freshness. Full nutritional content and biological absorption is exactly what you need in a food or super-food supplement. Don't be fooled by other companies saying products grown outside the USA are superior. Products imported from India, Brazil, Philippines, and other countries are far less expensive for these companies, but lack nutritional integrity.

Companies import to save money and use marketing to twist he truth to help support their bottom line. At Moringa Heath sayings like "you get what you pay for", and "the proof is in the pudding" could never ring more true. Your results are our best testimony.

You don't have to be a botanist to know the difference. Often simple visual comparisons can be evidence of temperature fluctuations in international transport, government enforced radiation, inappropriate drying and common heat induced friction processing techniques, leave little to no nutritional value in cheep imported products. Further concern is that these ingredients are being put inside tea bags, rice flower infused capsules,

and varied other products where your naked eye cannot discern
even the most basic quality test.

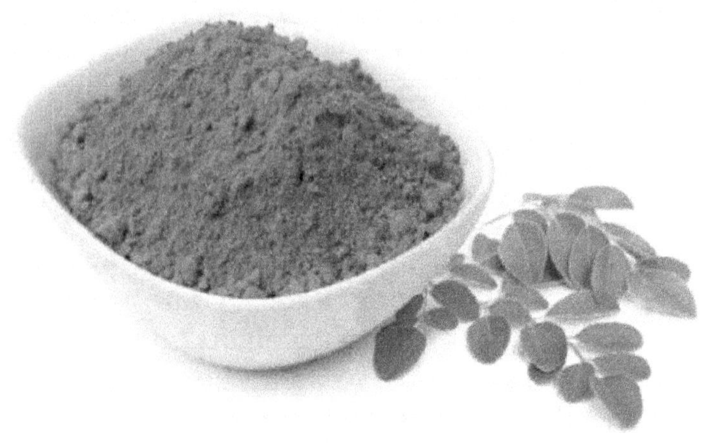

Moringa Health only uses the finest pure Moringa cultivated
through many years of cross breeding, and pain staking attention
to detail from soil quality through to proprietary processing. We
use sophisticated testing equipment to ensure the highest quality throughout all our product line be it powders or oils. It is essential that Moringa is dried at a specific constant humidity level
and that the drying process is prolonged for a 72 hour period.

Many companies boast their "specialized" flash drying process.
Cost reducing flash drying kills nutritional value and the benefits
of Moringa. Grinding and other forms of processing create friction heat and further degrade the nutritional value. At Moringa
Health we use proprietary systems with forced air to powderize

our leaf, as we take your health, the health of your family, and our families very seriously and are committed to the finest quality.

Though we offer hands down the finest pure Moringa, oil, leaves and seed in the world we also are famous for our moringa based rain forest infused botanical formulations. The formulations you will find here are specifically meant to change people lives, and that is why we have some of the best re-order rates in the industry.

Moringa Health has a passion for world hunger and has sponsored a global food awareness initiative called Leaf Life. A portion of all of your purchases go to support the Leaf Life awareness initiative.

I hope you come away with a greater understanding of why Moringa Health products should be the one and only choice for you and your family.

MIRACLE BENEFITS

NUTRITIONAL DATA

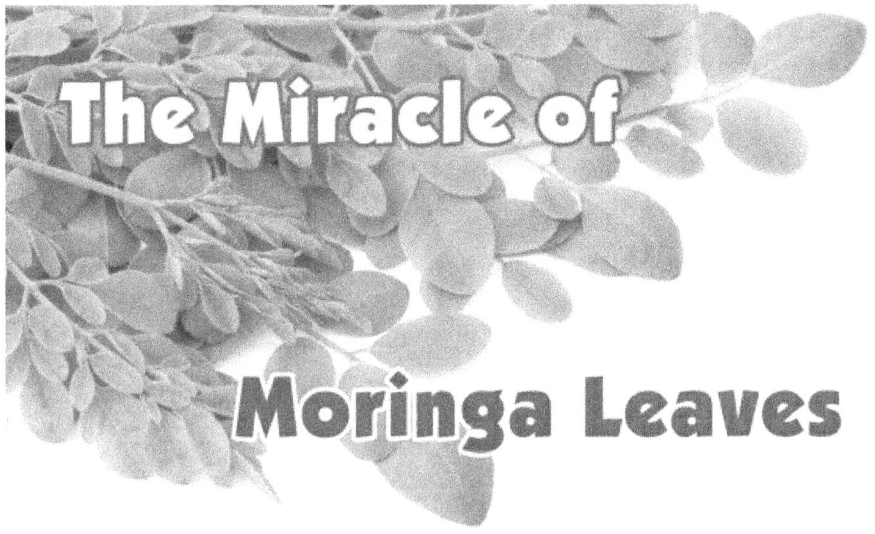

This remarkable tree has countless **health benefits**:

Pure properly processed and handled, Moringa Olifera improves immunity, improves blood stream, maintains blood sugar level, has anti-inflammatory properties, anti-aging properties, strengthens mental health, increases energy etc, etc.. It also contains anti-cancer compounds which prevent cancer cells from growing and spreading, these compounds are especially effective in against cancer. Moringa will cleanse your liver as well. An interesting fact is that when this tree's seeds crack, they cleanse polluted water. It has been proven that they reduce water's blurry state and cleans it from bacteria and clay. Yes you heard that correct Moringa seeds will make unpalatable water palatable.

In Exodus 15:25 in the holey bible it says speaks of a tree like this, "use the tree to purify the water". 25 So Moses cried out to the Lord for help, and the Lord showed him a piece of wood. Moses threw it into the water, and this made the water good to drink.

Moringa's primary health benefits are "hidden" in its leaves' nutrient value. In one dose of this tree's leaves you will find:

- 125% of the daily dose of calcium
- 61% of daily dose of magnesium
- 41% of daily dose of potassium
- 71% of daily dose of iron
- 272% of daily dose of vitamin A
- 22% of daily dose of vitamin C

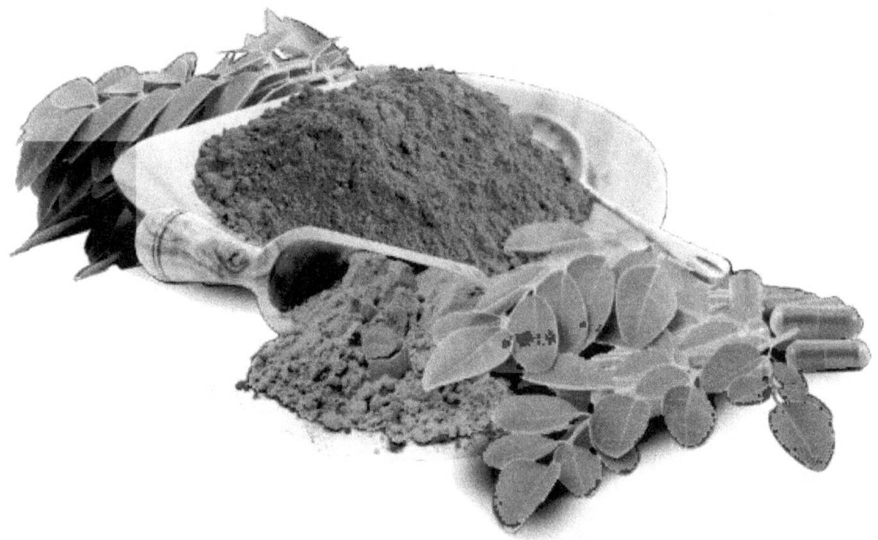

There is no other **"super food"** on the planet with this kind of supply. Moringa is completely healthy product that not only provides nutrients, but also improves the overall health of people of any age or race.

Young fruits of this tree are highly valued. They can be eaten raw or be prepared the same as green beans or peas. Fully grown fruits, on the other hand, are eaten fried and taste like peanuts.

The fruits have about 40% of oil ingredients which are used to produce cooking oil, also known as Ben oil, which is very similar to olive oil. The leaves are used as vegetables in salads. Moringa's fruit's peel can be used as a sunscreen lotion and the flowers, which are rich in potassium and calcium, can be used as foods.

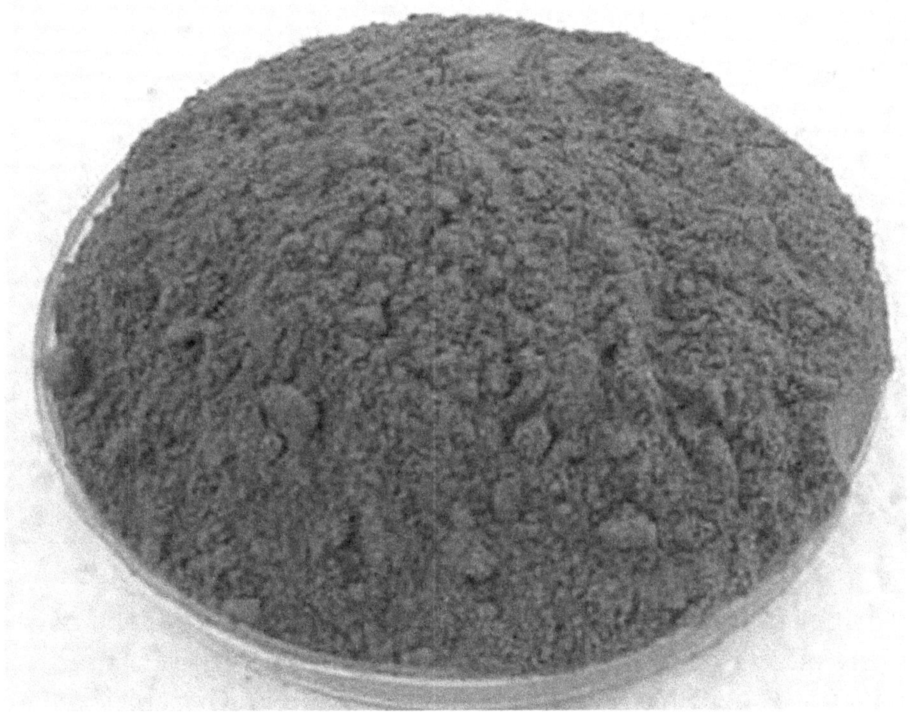

The Moringa tree can grow from 10 to 15 meters in height and in good environment it can live up to 20 years. People who grow this tree cut only 1, 5 meters of tree's branches in order to collect its leaves and fruits. All parts of this tree are edible and have healing properties, including the leaves, flowers, root and seeds.

This tree was used as a healing herb for the first time 1000 years ago. The proof of this, however, was discovered in the end of 1940. Indian scientists indentified Moringa's active ingredient which has antibacterial properties. Here are some of its amazing properties as shown in the world's leading health and medical journals:

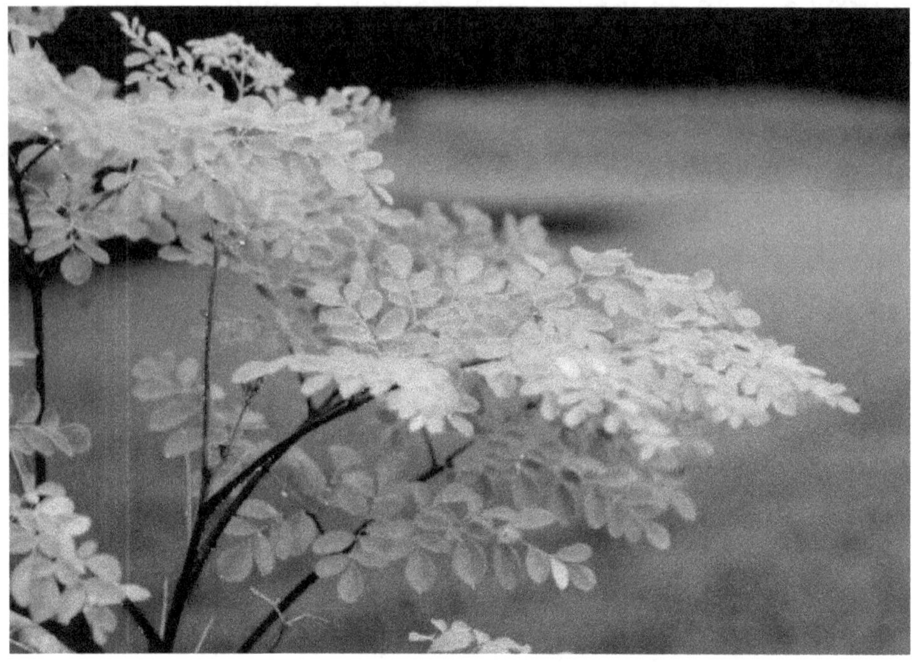

Moringa blocks cancer cells by protecting them from the damaging effects of powerful chemical toxins. Moringa is used to benefit the health of people challenged by ulcerative colitis. "Results show that a combination of Moringa oleifera root extracts with C. sinensis fruit rind extract is effective in the treatment of UC and results are comparable with the standard drug prednisolone." Moringa protects the liver against chemical toxins so it functions optimally.

Moringa also restores antioxidant activity to the liver by preventing early injury. Protects against experimental diabetes. "In conclusion, M. oleifera exerts protective effects against STZ-induced diabetes. The MOMtE exhibited significant anti-diabetic and antioxidant activity and active constituents may be isolated from the extract for evaluation in future clinical studies." These findings support the traditional usage of M. oleifera extracts for wound healing.

Moringa Oleifera is a species of tree native to the Himalayan Mountains of Northern India, and Southeast Asia, Africa and South America. Now cultivated, and perfected in the good old USA; non-radiated pure, and packed with fresh nutrients by Moringa Health! With a full spectrum of nutrients, Moringa Oleifera is the most nutrient-dense plant ever studied. Moringa leaf powder is a natural plant product for general health that promotes cardiovascular, neurological, prostate, vision health, proper digestion, energy and a normal healthy immune system support.

Moringa leaf provides antioxidants, proteins, vitamins, amino acids, flavonoids, fibers, minerals, chlorophyll, beta carotene and phenols benefits. Moringa has more than 90 essential nutrition compounds. Moringa Health's Moringa Oleifera is grown in the USA- The most nutritious plant ever studied, contains two important classes of compounds:

The Vitamin Content of Moringa Oleifera

Moringa oleifera is **rich with diverse vitamins, minerals, and amino acids.** Best of all, these nutrients are readily available for your body to use. The great majority of multivitamins available in the supermarket today are created in laboratories, where ingredients are synthesized and packed into a small pill. Unfortunately, most of these ingredients are not easily absorbed by the body because they are not sourced from whole foods. Moringa is a natural, whole-food source for vitamins, minerals, protein, antioxidants, and other important compounds that your body relies on to stay healthy. A single Moringa capsule contains a full spectrum of nutrients.

Moringa benefits are derived from the plant's high concentration of bio-available nutrients. It contains high levels of Vitamin A (beta carotene), Vitamin B1 (Thiamine), Vitamin B2 (Riboflavin), Vitamin B3 (Niacin), Vitamin B6 (Pyridoxine), Vitamin B7 (Biotin), Vitamin C (Ascorbic Acid), Vitamin D (Cholecalciferol), Vitamin E (Tocopherol) and Vitamin K.

Vitamin A (beta carotene) is needed by the retina of the eye in the form of a specific metabolite, the light-absorbing molecule retinal. This molecule is absolutely necessary for both scotopic vision and color vision. Vitamin A also functions in a very different role - as an irreversibly oxidized form retinoic acid, which is an important hormone-like growth factor for epithelial and other cells.

Vitamin B1 (thiamine) helps fuel the body by converting blood sugar into energy. It keeps the mucous membranes healthy and is essential for the nervous system and cardiovascular and muscular functions.

Vitamin B2 (riboflavin) is required for a wide variety of cellular processes. Like the other B vitamins, it plays a key role in energy metabolism, and for the metabolism of fats, ketone bodies, carbohydrates, and proteins. It is the central component of the cofactors FAD and FMN, and is therefore required by all "Flavoproteins".

Vitamin B3 (niacin), like all B complex vitamins, is necessary for healthy skin, hair, eyes, and liver. It also helps the nervous system function properly. Niacin helps the body produce sex and stress-related hormones in the adrenal glands and other parts of the body. It is effective in improving circulation and reducing cholesterol levels in the blood.

Vitamin B6 (pyridoxine) is required for the synthesis of the neurotransmitters serotonin and norepinephrine and for myelin formation. Pyridoxine deficiency in adults principally affects the peripheral nerves, skin, mucous membranes, and the blood cell system. In children, the central nervous system (CNS) is also affected. Deficiency can occur in people with uremia, alcoholism, cirrhosis, hyperthyroidism, malabsorption syndromes, congestive heart failure (CHF), and in those taking certain medications.

Vitamin B7 (biotin) has vital metabolic functions. Without biotin as a co-factor, many enzymes do not work properly, and serious complications can occur, including varied diseases of the skin, intestinal tract, and nervous system.

Biotin can help address high blood glucose levels in people with type 2 diabetes, and is helpful in maintaining healthy hair and nails, decreasing insulin resistance and improving glucose tolerance, and possibly preventing birth defects. It plays a role in energy metabolism, and has been used to treat alopecia, cancer, Crohn's disease, hair loss, Parkinson's disease, peripheral neuropathy, Rett syndrome, seborrheic dermatitis, and vaginal candidiasis.

Vitamin C (ascorbic acid) is one of the safest and most effective nutrients, experts say. It may not be the cure for the common cold (though it's thought to help prevent more serious complications), but the benefits of vitamin C may include protection against immune system deficiencies, cardiovascular disease, prenatal health problems, eye disease, and wrinkles.

Vitamin D (cholecalciferol) is essential for promoting calcium absorption in the gut and maintaining adequate serum calcium and phosphate concentrations to enable normal mineralization of bone and prevent hypocalcemic tetany. It is also needed for bone growth and bone remodeling by osteoblasts and osteoclasts. Without sufficient vitamin D, bones can become thin, brittle, or misshapen. Vitamin D sufficiency prevents rickets in children and osteomalacia in adults. Together with calcium, vitamin D also helps protect the elderly from osteoporosis. Vitamin D has other roles in human health, including modulation of neuromuscular and immune function and reduction of inflammation.

Vitamin E describes a family of eight antioxidants, four tocopherols and four tocotrienols. alpha-tocopherol (a-tocopherol) is the only form of vitamin E that is actively maintained in the human body and is therefore, the form of vitamin E found in the largest quantities in the blood and tissue. Vitamin E, a fat-soluble vitamin, protects vitamin A and essential fatty acids from oxidation in the body cells and prevents breakdown of body tissues.

Vitamin K is needed for blood to properly clot, and for the liver to make blood clotting factors, including factor II (prothrombin), factor VII (proconvertin), factor IX (thromboplastin component), and factor X (Stuart factor). Other clotting factors that depend on vitamin K are protein C, protein S, and protein Z. Deficiency of vitamin K or disturbances of liver function (for example, severe liver failure) may lead to deficiencies of clotting factors and excess bleeding.

Amino Acids: The Foundation of Our Body

There are 18 different amino acids, or protein types, that are the building blocks for a healthy body. Non-essential amino acids are proteins that the body can synthesize by itself, provided there is enough nitrogen, carbon, hydrogen, and oxygen available. Essential amino acids are proteins supplied by the food you eat. They must be consumed in your diet as the human body either cannot make them or cannot make them in sufficient quantities to meet your body's needs.

Proteins act as enzymes, hormones, and antibodies for your immune system. They maintain fluid balance and keep the levels of acid and alkalinity in check. Proteins also transport substances such as oxygen, vitamins, and minerals to target cells throughout the body. Structural proteins, such as collagen and keratin, are responsible for the formation of bones, teeth, hair, and the outer layer of skin and they help maintain the structure of blood vessels and other tissues.

Enzymes are proteins that facilitate chemical reactions without being changed in the process. Hormones (chemical messengers) are proteins that travel to one or more specific target tissues or organs, and many have important regulatory functions. Insulin, for example, plays a key role in regulating the amount of glucose in the blood.

The human body also uses protein to manufacture antibodies (giant protein molecules), which combat invading antigens. Antigens are usually foreign substances such as bacteria and viruses that have entered the body and could potentially be harmful. Immunoproteins, also called immunoglobulins or antibodies, defend your body from possible attack from these invaders by binding to the antigens and inactivation them.

If these critical components for a healthy body are not provided as part of a healthy diet, your body will look for other sources for them. This can include the breakdown of your organs, leading to chronic problems such as liver and kidney problems, diabetes, and heart disease.

Moringa Oleifera Leaf Powder

It contains all of the essential amino acids required for a healthy body. Dried Moringa leaf is a nutritional powerhouse and contains all of the following amino acids.

ISOLEUCINE builds proteins and enzymes and it provides ingredients used to create other essential biochemical components in the body, some of which promote energy and stimulate the brain to maintain state of alertness.

LEUCINE works with isoleucine to build proteins and enzymes which enhance the body's energy and alertness.

LYSINE ensures your body absorbs the right amount of calcium. It also helps form collagen used in bone cartilage and connective tissues. In addition, lysine aids in the production of antibodies, hormones, and enzymes. Recent studies have shown lysine improves the balance of nutrients that reduce viral growth.

METHIONINE primarily supplies sulfur to your body. It is known to prevent hair, skin, and nail problems, while lowering cholesterol levels as it increases the liver's production of lecithin. Methionine reduces liver fat and protects the kidneys, which reduces bladder irritation.

PHENYLALAINE produces the chemical needed to transmit signals between nerve cells and the brain. It can help with concentration and alertness, reduce hunger pains, and improve memory and mood.

THREONINE is an important part of collagen, elastin, and enamel proteins. It assists metabolism and helps prevent fat build-up in the liver while boosting the body's digestive and intestinal tracts.

TRYPTOPHAN supports the immune system, alleviates insomnia, and reduces anxiety, depression, and the symptoms of migraine headaches. It also is beneficial in decreasing the risk of artery and heart spasms as it works with lysine to reduce cholesterol levels.

VALINE is important in promoting a sharp mind, coordinated muscles, and a calm mood.

Non-Essential Amino Acids in Moringa

ALANINE is important for energy in muscle tissue, brain, and central nervous system. It strengthens the immune system by producing antibodies. Alanine also helps in the healthy metabolism of sugars and organic acids in the body.

ARGININE causes the release of the growth hormones considered crucial for optimal muscle growth and tissue repair. It also improves immune responses to bacteria, viruses, and tumor cells while promoting the healing of the body's wounds.

ASPARTIC ACID helps rid the body of ammonia created by cellular waste. When the ammonia enters the circulatory system it can act as a highly toxic substance which can damage the central nervous system. Recent studies have also shown that aspartic acid may decrease fatigue and increase endurance.

CYSTINE functions as an antioxidant and is a powerful aid to the body in protecting against radiation and pollution. It can help slow the aging process, deactivate free radicals, and neutralize toxins. It also helps in protein synthesis and presents cellular change. It is necessary for the formation of new skin cells, which aids in the recovery from burns and surgical operations.

GLUTAMIC ACID is food for the brain. It improves mental capacities, helps speed the healing of ulcers, reduces fatigue, and curbs sugar cravings.

GLYCINE promotes the release of oxygen required in the cell-making process. It is also important in the manufacturing of hormones responsible for a strong immune system

HISTIDINE is used in the treatment of rheumatoid arthritis, allergies, ulcers, and anemia. A lack of histidine may lead to poor hearing.

SERINE is important in storing glucose in the liver and muscles. Its antibodies help strengthen the body's immune system. Plus, it synthesizes fatty acid sheaths around nerve fibers.

PROLINE is extremely important for the proper function of your joints and tendons. It also helps maintain and strengthen heart muscles.

TYROSINE transmits nerve impulses to your brain. It helps overcome depression; improves memory; increases mental alertness; plus promotes the healthy functioning of the thyroid, adrenal, and pituitary glands.

an Exhaustive List:

Antioxidants:

- Vitamin A
- Vitamin C
- Vitamin E
- Vitamin K
- Vitamin B (Choline)
- Vitamin B1 (Thiamin)
- Vitamin B2 (Riboflavin)
- Vitamin B3 (Niacin)
- Vitamin B6
- Alanine
- Alpha-Carotene
- Arginine
- Beta-Carotene
- Beta-sitosterol
- Caffeoyquinic Acid
- Campesterol
- Cartenoids
- Chlorophyll
- Chromium
- Delta-5-Avenasterol
- Delta-7- Avenasterol
- Glutathione
- Histidine
- Indole Acetic Acid
- Indoleacetonitrile
- Kaempferal
- Leucine
- Lutein
- Methionine
- Myristic-Acid

- Palmitic-Acid
- Prolamine
- Proline
- Quercetin
- Rutin
- Selenium
- Threonine
- Tryptophan
- Xanthins
- Xanthophyll
- Zeatin
- Zeaxanthin
- Zinc

Anti-Inflammatories:

- Vitamin A
- Vitamin B1 (Thiamin)
- Vitamin C
- Vitamin E
- Arginine
- Beta-sitosterol
- Caffeolquinic Acid
- Calcium
- Chlorophyll
- Copper
- Cystine
- Omega 3
- Omega 6
- Omega 9
- Fiber
- Glutathione

- Histidine
- Indole Acetic Acid
- Indoleacetonitrile
- Isoleucine
- Kaempferal
- Leucine
- Magnesium
- Oleic Acid
- Phenylalanine
- Potassium
- Quercetin
- Rutin
- Selenium
- Stigmasterol
- Sulfur
- Tryptophan
- Tyrosine
- Zeatin
- Zinc

Here is some Typical Nutritional Data

____

Macronutrients (per 100g)
- Moisture (%)   7.5
- Calories   205
- Protein (g)   27.1
- Fat (g)   2.3

- Carbohydrates (g)   38.2
- Fiber (g)   19.2

Amino acids (g/16gN)

- Arginine   1.33
- Histidine   0.61
- Isoleucine   1.32
- Leucine   1.95
- Lysine   1.32
- Methionine   0.35
- Phenylalinine   1.39
- Threonine   1.19
- Tryptophan   0.43
- Valine   1.06

Minerals (per 100g)

- Calcium (mg)   2003
- Magnesium (mg)   368
- Phosporous (mg)   204
- Potassium (mg)   1324
- Copper (mg)   19.1
- Iron (mg)   28.2
- Zinc (mg)   3.29

Vitamins (mg per 100g)

- Vitamin A - Beta Carotene   16.3
- Vitamin B1 - Thiamin (mg)   2.6
- Vitamin B2 - Riboflavin (mg)   20.5
- Vitamin B3 - Nicotinic acid (mg)   8.2
- Vitamin C - Ascorbic acid (mg)   17.3
- Vitamin E – Tocopherol acetate (mg)   113.0

Physical Characteristics

- Appearance   Powder

- Color   Rich green
- Flavor   Tart

Allergens

Our product is free of milk, eggs, fish, Crustacean shellfish, tree nuts, peanuts, wheat, soybeans and is gluten-free.

How does Moringa stand up to other organic options?

When yougo to the market you probable would never consider leaving out the fruits and veggies. Especially not the leafy greens.

LETS COMPARE:

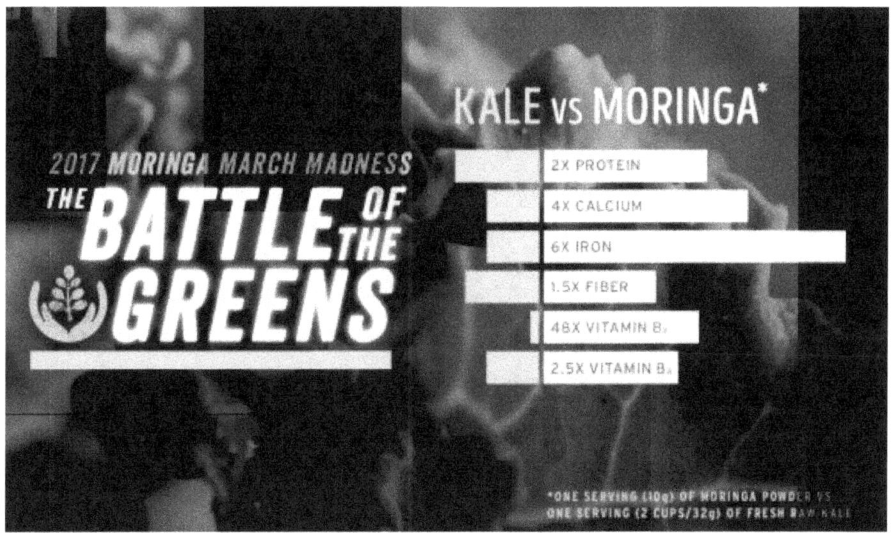

	Moringa Leaves - Raw (100g)	Kale - Raw (100g)
Riboflavin (mg)	0.66	0.13
Vitamin B-6 (mg)	1.2	0.27
Iron (mg)	4	1.47
Thiamine (mg)	0.26	0.11
Niacin (mg)	2.2	1
Protein (g)	9.4	4.3
Calcium (mg)	185	150
Vitamin A (IU)	7564	9990
Potassium (mg)	337	491
Fiber (g)	2	3.6
Vitamin C (mg)	51.7	120

Battle of the Greens!

Round Three

Collard Greens   **Moringa Leaves**
mean of 100g

Collard Greens		Moringa Leaves
3 g	**Protein** — An egg has about 6g protein while a steak has about 77g.	9.4 g
232 mg	**Calcium** — Your teeth and bones will thank you.	185 mg
0.47 mg	**Iron** — Iron deficiency anemia; the most common nutrient deficiency in the world.	4 mg
4 g	**Fiber** — Recommended daily intake is 20-35g. Keep those bowels moving!	2 g
5019 IU	**Vitamin A** — Maintain your good vision, healthy skin, teeth, and other skeletal and soft tissues.	7564 IU
0.05 mg	**Thiamine B1** — Also vitamin B1; deficiency of this vitamin can lead to brain death!	0.26 mg
0.13 mg	**Riboflavin B2** — Also vitamin B2; necessary to replenish the body's red blood cells	0.66 mg
0.74 mg	**Niacin B3** — Also vitamin B3; used to treat high cholestrol, diabetes, and some skin conditions.	2.2 mg
0.17 mg	**Vitamin B6** — Regulates blood sugar and creates the body's hemoglobin and antibodies.	1.2 mg
213 mg	**Potassium** — Mineral and electrolyte that helps muscle recovery post-workout.	337 mg

Score 2   **Moringa Wins!**   Score 9

Battle of the Greens!

Moringa vs Spirulina

Moringa		Spirulina
	Protein	
2.7 g	An egg has about 6g protein while a steak has about 77.	5.75g
	Calcium	
174 mg	Your teeth and bones will thank you.	12 mg
	Iron	
15.8 mg	Iron anemia: the most common nutrient deficiency in the world.	2.85 mg
	Fiber	
3.3 g	Recommended daily intake is 20-35g. Keep those bowels moving!	0.36 g
	Vitamin A	
910 iu	Maintain your good vision, healthy skin, teeth, and other skeletal and soft tissues.	57 iu
	Vitamin C	
0.99 mg	Power your immune system! Fend off sickness!	1.01 mg
	Potassium	
140 mg	Mineral and electrolyte that helps muscle recovery post-workout.	136.3 mg
	Carbohydrate	
5.1 g	The main source of energy for our bodies.	2.39 g
	Sodium	
2 mg	Many Americans consume far too much.	105 mg
	Calories	
35	Shoot for more nutrients with fewer calories.	29

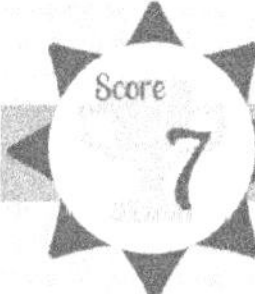

Battle of the Greens!

Spinach Leaves

Moringa Leaves
mean of 100g

	Spinach Leaves	Moringa Leaves
Protein — An egg has about 6g protein while a steak has about 77g.	2.9 g	9.4 g
Calcium — Your teeth and bones will thank you.	99 mg	185 mg
Iron — Iron deficiency anemia: the most common nutrient deficiency in the world.	2.7 mg	4 mg
Fiber — Recommended daily intake is 20-35g. Keep those bowels moving!	2.2 g	2.0 g
Vitamin A — Maintain your good vision, healthy skin, teeth, and other skeletal and soft tissues.	9377 IU	7564 IU
Thiamine B1 — Also vitamin B1; deficiency of this vitamin can lead to brain death!	0.08 mg	0.26 mg
Riboflavin B2 — Also vitamin B2; necessary to replenish the body's red blood cells.	0.19 mg	0.66 mg
Niacin B3 — Also vitamin B3; used to treat high cholestrol, diabetes, and some skin conditions.	0.72 mg	2.2 mg
Vitamin B6 — Regulates blood sugar and creates the body's hemoglobin and antibodies.	0.20 mg	1.2 mg
Vitamin C — Power your immune system! Fend off sickness!	28 mg	51.7 mg
Potassium — Mineral and electrolyte that helps muscle recovery post-workout.	558 mg	337 mg

Score 3

Moringa Wins!

Score 8

Battle of the Greens!

Swiss Chard | Moringa Leaves
mean of 100g

Swiss Chard		Moringa Leaves
1.8 g	**Protein** An egg has about 6g protein while a steak has about 77g.	9.4 g
51 mg	**Calcium** Your teeth and bones will thank you.	185 mg
1.8 mg	**Iron** Iron deficiency anemia: the most common nutrient deficiency in the world.	4 mg
1.6 g	**Fiber** Recommended daily intake is 20-35g. Keep those bowels moving!	2 g
6116 IU	**Vitamin A** Maintain your good vision, healthy skin, teeth, and other skeletal and soft tissues.	7564 IU
0.04 mg	**Thiamine B1** Also vitamin B1; deficiency of this vitamin can lead to brain death!	0.26 mg
0.09 mg	**Riboflavin B2** Also vitamin B2; necessary to replenish the body's red blood cells.	0.66 mg
0.4 mg	**Niacin B3** Also vitamin B3; used to treat high cholestrol, diabetes, and some skin conditions.	2.2 mg
0.09 mg	**Vitamin B6** Regulates blood sugar and creates the body's hemoglobin and antibodies.	1.2 mg
30 mg	**Vitamin C** Power your immune system! Fend off sickness!	51.7 mg
379 mg	**Potassium** Mineral and electrolyte that helps muscle recovery post-workout.	337 mg

Score 1 — Moringa Wins! — **Score 10**

Battle of the Greens!

Matcha Powder
Moringa Powder

mean of 100g

	Matcha Powder		Moringa Powder
357 cal	**Calories** ...a close call		375 cal
72.6 g	**Carbohydrate** The main source of energy for our bodies.		50 g
10.2 g	**Fiber** Recommended daily intake is 20-35g!		25 g
7.3 g	**Protein** An egg contains ~6g protein while a steak ~77g.		37.5 g
94.2 mg	**Calcium** Your bones will thank you.		2000 mg
2.2 mg	**Sodium** Excess sodium affects the heart and kidneys!		12.5 mg
2.8 mg	**Iron** Iron deficiency anemia: the most common nutrient deficiencies in the world.		31.3 mg
511 µg	**Vitamin A** For your eyes and a healthy immune system!		63k µg
42 mg	**Vitamin C** Power your immune system! Fend off sickness!		175 mg
8.7 mg	**Vitamin E** A powerful antioxidant to protect your body.		112.5 mg

Score 3 — Moringa Wins! — **Score 7**

	Moringa Leaves - Raw (100g)	Kale - Raw (100g)
Riboflavin (mg)	0.66	0.13
Vitamin B-6 (mg)	1.2	0.27
Iron (mg)	4	1.47
Thiamine (mg)	0.26	0.11
Niacin (mg)	2.2	1
Protein (g)	9.4	4.3
Calcium (mg)	185	150
Vitamin A (IU)	7564	9990
Potassium (mg)	337	491
Fiber (g)	2	3.6
Vitamin C (mg)	51.7	120

Check Out That Vitamin C

Battle of the Greens!

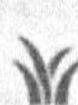 

Round Eight

Moringa	vs	Wheatgrass

Protein
2.7g — Build strong muscles! (Too close to call) — 2.5g

Calcium
174mg — Your teeth and bones will thank you. — 37.5mg

Iron
15.8mg — Iron anemia: the most common nutrient deficiency in the world. — 2mg

Vitamin A
901 iu — Maintain your good vision, healthy skin, teeth, and other skeletal and soft tissues. — 4,750 iu

Vitamin C
0.99mg — Necessary for the growth, development and repair of all body tissues. — 17.5mg

Vitamin K
147 mcg — Essential to blood clotting and building strong bones. — 100mcg

Fiber
3.3g — Recommended daily intake is 20-35g. Keep those bowels moving! — 2.5g

Potassium
140mg — Aids nerve conduction and muscle contraction... plays a role in every heartbeat! — 287.5mg

Calories
35 — Shoot for more nutrients with fewer calories. — 43.75

Sodium
2g — Nearly 1/3 Americans have high blood pressure; keep salt intake low — 2.5g

Carbs
5.1g — Keep those energy levels up! (Too close to call) — 5g

Score 6 — Moringa Wins — **Score 3**

Moringa And Global Hunger

Moringa is a fast growing tree which can reach a maximum high of 6-14m and a diameter of 2-4m and can help feed many starving children and familes around the world.. How can "Moringa Tree" help solve malnutrition globally? Malnutrition is a significant factor in many countries around the world. People suffer the fate of lack of food and nutrients. Particularly children are suffering and dying at record rates across the globe. In the poorest countries one child out of five will die before the age of 5 (can you imagine?). Many millions of people die from chronic malnutrition. Here we can find several factors such as: arid climate, drought, poverty, unemployment, war, refugees…etc. Moringa grows wild in many parts of the world. Moringa Health and other companies are working together to create a global hunger awareness campaign by growing trees to stop this global starvation and malnutrition epidemic.

Moringa grows quickly from seeds or cuttings and generates itself after severe pruning. The tree is often cultivated as a fence around the house or garden. The tree is known for its many medicinal uses. Moringa parts and their uses:

Seeds (kernels, shells, oil, fuel, cooking, cosmetic, medicinal and industrial uses, animal feed, water purification)
Roots (medicinal use, human consumption)
Bark (medicinal use)
Leaves (human consumption, medicinal use, animal feed)
Stems (animal feed)
Twigs (animal feed)
Root and branches (fertilizer)

The Seeds
The seed powder and oil produced from the seed pods of the

"Moringa Tree" can help to purify water of muds, bacteria and viruses. So the seed and oil therefore can help digestive and gut issues. Moringa seeds contain more than 30-45% oil. In the cosmetic industry, in the soap industry, in the fine machinery and in the perfume industry. The oil contains plenty of oleic acid (69-74%). Other edible oils contain only about 39-41% oleic acid. The press-cake as a by product of the oil extraction process is comprised of a very high level of protein that can be eaten. The dry seeds can be ground to a powder and can be used in different sauces. The seeds can also be good in salads.

Leaves:
After cutting the trees the leaves are then washed and removed and stripped from the branches. Damaged leaves are discarded. After this they are brought into the drying room. The drying room is a ventilated room. It's important to dry the leaves in 2-3 days, depending on conditions of humidity. Traditionally companies after drying the leaves are pounded in a mortar in a groundnut mill or in a hammer mill to pack it into a clean cardboard with polythene bag and heat-sealed that the powder in the box is hermetically sealed. Moringa Health uses a patented screen blowing process for friction free refining to help retain the nutritional integrity. This is important for freshness quality. The Vitamin C content and other vitamins as well are very high in the moringa leaves. Fresh and very young leaves can be eaten raw and taste great similar to pepper.

Nutritional values
(100gr.) fresh Moringa leaves:
Proteins
5-7 grams

Minerals
Calcium (CA)
360-560 mg
Potassium (K)

200-500 mg
Magnesium (Mg)
80-120 mg
Phosphorus (P)
50-120 mg
Iron (Fe)
5-8 mg
Manganese (Mn)
1,2-2,6 mg
Copper (Cu)
0,2-0,3 mg

Vitamins
Vitamin C
120-220 mg
Vitamin A
1500-4000 mg
Vitamin E
150-200 mg
100 grams of fresh Moringa leaves could cover 100% of daily need. Important is that the fresh leaves are not heated as the vitamin A is destroyed.

Stems and Twigs: Have a low crude protein content as well.

Chapter 4

KING OF SUPER FOODS

ORGANIC POWDER

Organic Moringa Health powder not only deserves inclusion, in the superfoods category, but is the undeniable, uncontestable raining KING because of the extensive health benefits it provides.

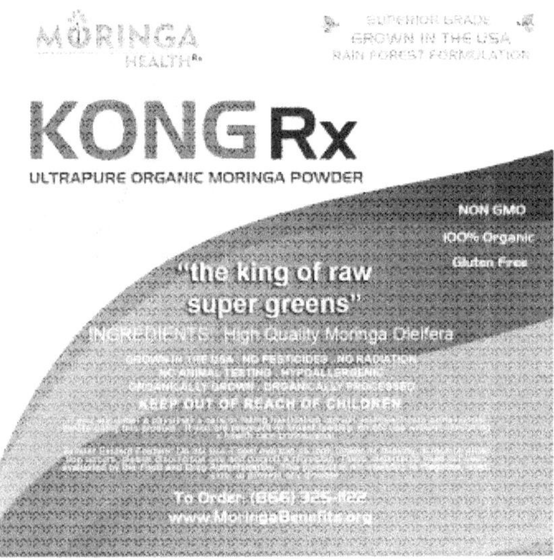

Those benefits include supporting health bones, regulating blood sugar, helping your skin maintain a youthful appearance, lowering cholesterol and helping control blood pressure. It is essential for you to maintain a healthy immune system so that your body can fight off infections and illnesses. Organic Moringa powder is revered for its immune-boosting quality. There is anecdotal evidence that this amazing powder can also aid in the prevention of cancer.

Organic moringa powder is a supplement that can enhance your overall well-being by boosting your energy level, increasing your stamina and improving your ability to concentrate, and continued use will enhance cognitive ability.

In order to give your body the support it needs to function at its best, you may want to make organic moringa powder bulk purchases.

We don't blame you!

This supplement can be a key factor in helping you achieve and remain committed to a <u>healthy lifestyle</u>. If you have chosen a vegan or vegetarian lifestyle, adding organic moringa leaf powder to your daily health regimen is a good way to get the protein you need to support muscle mass. It can help detoxify your body, keep you from feeling sluggish and relieve feelings of depression and anxiety. This powder can help prevent hair loss, stimulate hair growth and support healthy vision and teeth.

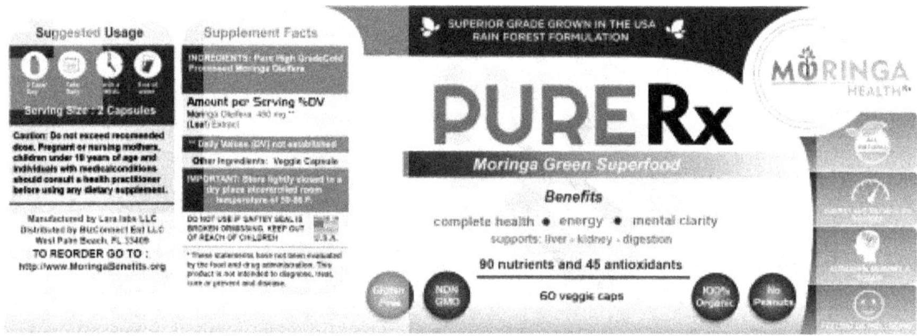

Uses of Moringa Powder

Athletes can use Moringa powder to help boost their energy level, build muscle mass and increase their endurance. Since this powder helps improve concentration, someone in college or someone whose job requires a lot of concentration could benefit from taking this powder. You can take it according to the time of day that you need it most based on when you experience an energy slump or when your concentration level drops. You can use this powder to detoxify your body. In addition to adding this powder to drinks, smoothies or almost any type of recipe so that it is consumed internally, you can also use

Moringa powder externally to gain an entirely different type of benefits. You can make a paste using Moringa powder and apply it to your skin to help keep it smooth and youthful-looking. Due to its healing benefits, Moringa powder can be applied directly to cuts or wounds to expedite healing.

Dosage

When you first begin using Organic Moringa leaf powder, it is recommended that you start with a ½ teaspoon per day (or more conveniently) 2 capsules a day. Keep in mind that Moringa Health's Moringa is much more potent than other internet or store bought Moringa, so you need much less. After taking this amount for a week, you can increase the dosage to 1 teaspoon or (4 capsules) then on up to 1 tablespoon per day so that you can take full advantage of the many benefits this powder provides. The total daily dosage does not have to be taken all at one time or at any specific time of day. The powder can be added to almost anything. However, when adding it to soups, stews or cooked dishes, it's best to add it at the end of cooking. This assures that you get the most nutritional value from the powder. Like with any herb everybody reacts differently, it is always a good idea to start slow.

Organic Moringa Powder for Diabetes

Organic Moringa powder provides **health benefits** that directly relate to issues that diabetics often face. Diabetics often have a compromised immune system. This powder supports a healthy immune system. Diabetics often have circulatory problems. Incorporating this powder into a diabetic-friendly diet can help prevent circulatory problems that are often caused by inflammation. Moringa powder can help maintain normal blood sugar levels. When levels are stabilized, many of the health concerns typically associated with diabetes do not occur. High blood sugar can lead to numerous other health problems. By helping balance insulin levels and possibly even lower blood sugar levels, Moringa powder can be a contributing factor in supporting the overall health of diabetics. Moringa specializes in repairing liver, and kidney function another reason it is essential for diabetics.

Side Effects

Generally, there are no side effects to Organic Moringa powder. Before you add any supplement to your diet, it is recommended that you consult with your physician to assure that it's safe for you. Note: Moringa seed is believed to be a strong libido enhancer, and restraint is advised. In addition, pure moringa powder can act as a laxative.

Storage and Shelf Life: Store in a cool, dry place. Shelf life: bags – up to 1 year. Bulk – up to 6 months.

UNIQUE FORMULATIONS

RAIN FOREST BLENDS

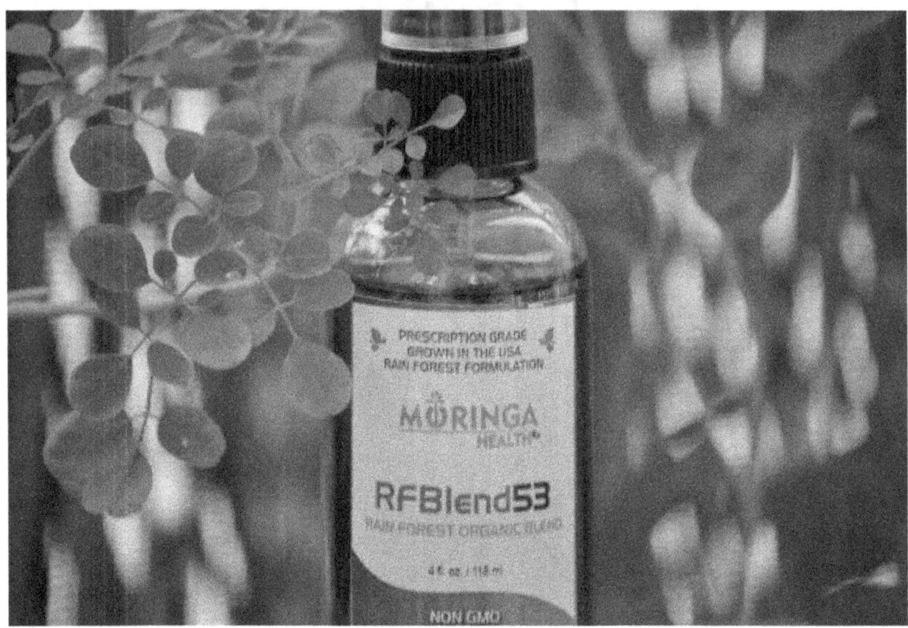

Moringa is a worldwide phenomenon as I mentioned before many countries populations use Moringa preventatively, and medicinally as a regularly daily part of their regimen. About 85% of the world population is ware of the benefits and many uses of Moringa oliefera. However, only about 6-7% of American knows about this incredible tree aid is benefits.

Currently there are about 8-9 companies that distribute moringa in the USA and it can be found in most cities from Whole Foods to Wal-Mart. However, "buyer beware" as these companies all import their Moringa form India, the Philippians and a variety of other countries. A handful import raw Moringa, and fill their capsules here and market it as "made in the USA".

Moringa Health is the only company that grows, processes, and manufactures in the USA. However, Moringa health takes it one important step further. We provide USA grown Moringa formulated with special rain forest herbal blends. These Moringa based formulations are a combination of the best Moringa in the world and closely guarded rain forest secrets handed down by traditional rain forest Shaman healers and herbal tribal specialist.

Moringa Health provides a variety of herbal Moringa formulations that target a variety of health conditions. respiratory system issues, cardiovascular, musculoskeletal, skin diseases, mental illness, digestive, neurological, urinary and reproductive, endocrine, as well as arthritis, cancer, aids, ADHD, PTSD, hepatitis, dementia, fibromyalgia, weight loss, seizure, and erectile dysfunction.

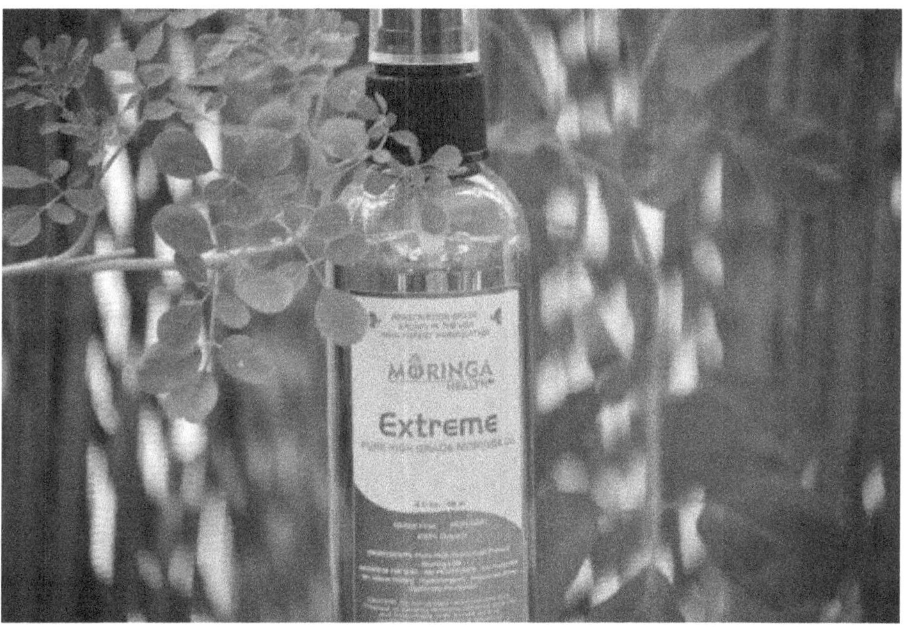

These **unique rain forest blends** combined with Moringa Health's first to market Moringa based CBD products have application for, drug rehab, pharmaceutical alternatives and reduction of use, massage therapy, physical therapy, chiropractic, wellness and anti-aging, intimacy aid, veteran herbal solutions, sports application, and more. We are very excited to offer these herbal solutions to the marketplace, and are most enthusiastic about hearing all of the remarkable stories form your customers and clients.

HEART FOR PEOPLE

MATTER OVER MONEY

Moringa Health has taken the position, and posture that our ideology will be that people are more important then profits. This fundamental principle is at the core of our company decisions, manufacturing and pricing. It is extremely more expensive to produce these quality products here in the USA than it is for other companies to place an order and import. But it is our goal to be steadfast and hold true to our principals and integrity from growing to marketing. When I say "matter over money" it simply means that people matter more to Moringa health than money does.

Compromise:

1. Process of mutual accommodation in which each party gives up something valuable, but without any party abandoning its claim or resorting to confrontation, hostilities, or litigation.
2. An unauthorized and weakening disclosure or modification of competitive, confidential, privileged, or proprietary information.

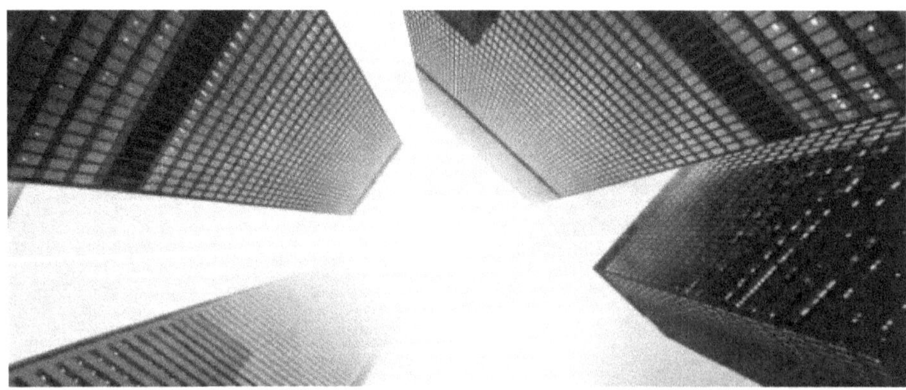

We are on a mission to provide health herbal alternatives to the general public without compromise. You know it is very interesting, while I was writing this I took a moment to Google "why businesses compromise", I was amazed as I could not find one article directly addressing this issue. It was as if it is a topic that no one wants to address, acknowledge or better yet admit.

I found this curious, as throughout the life of a company there are growing pressures and unlimited opportunity to compromise. Most of the time there is literally no choice companies can even take in the process. To be competitive and to survive from the very onset companies often have to levitate to follow suite in the decisions their competitors have taken. This may sound a bit cynical but the truth is accounting and the bottom line, often makes decision for companies where the directors have no say. Either there is a choice to do things the way everyone else is or simply decide not to start at all.

At Moringa Health we have been fortunate as money is not our principal directive. To give you an example of what I mean, I cannot specify companies here, but at one time we were offered several million dollars for the release of one of our formulations. The reason being is this large company tried to test our product, and steal the formulation. But when that failed they decide to take the high road and leverage us into disclosure. The reason they could not figure out the formulation is that some of our herbal formulations have been handed down form generations of rain forest secrets.

The formulation and some of the ingredients simply does not exist. However, we had to decline the generous offer. Simply because the relationships we share in the rain forest and the people who live there were is simply more important to us than money. It is this kind of ideology and principal that keeps us growing, and processing USA formulations for the general public. Moringa

Health will never compromise at the cost of integrity or at he cost of people.

 We are a people driven company and our products represent that ideology.

THE FIFTH PILLAR

ALTERNATIVE MEDICINE

At the core of every great company rests a vision that is greater and larger than what seems possible.

The current state of affairs is that as a western medical society we embrace a "pac" of wellness professionals as our go to resource of information for health. This "pac" includes those professionals we are all ready to embrace, and run to in time of need. The consortium includes, a medical doctor, physical therapist, chiropractor, nutritionist, and a physiatrist.

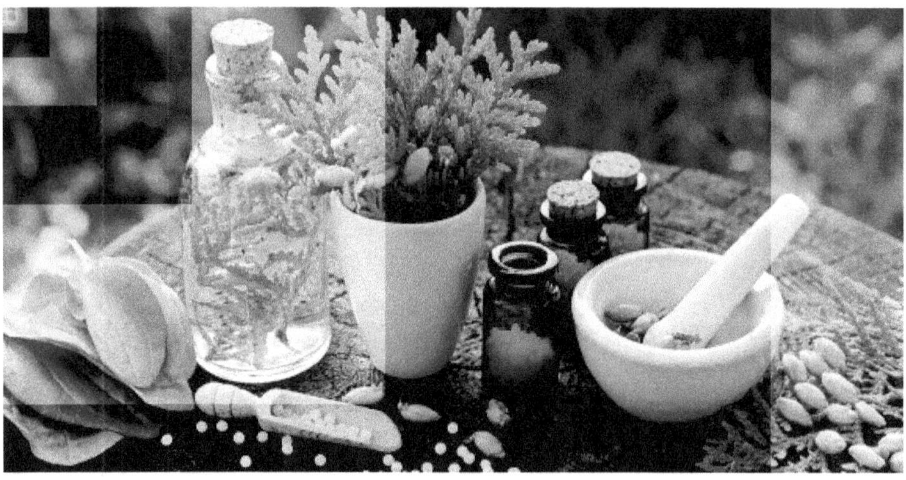

Ironically, there is one very important sixth cog in the wheel that is missing. Without this missing cog the wheel is not able to roll and leaves us off balance, and out of alignment. We all know that most pharmaceutical products are created, and sensitized form some form of plant extract. In this synthinization process the natural buffers in the plant are removed.

Pharmaceutical products deliver an **isolated solution** to a specific problem. However, because the natural buffers have been removed, these medicines leave us will a host of undesirable side effects. We are all much to familiar with the plethora of television commercials that have a never ending often ironic list of possible side affects, and on going disclaimers of prescribed use.

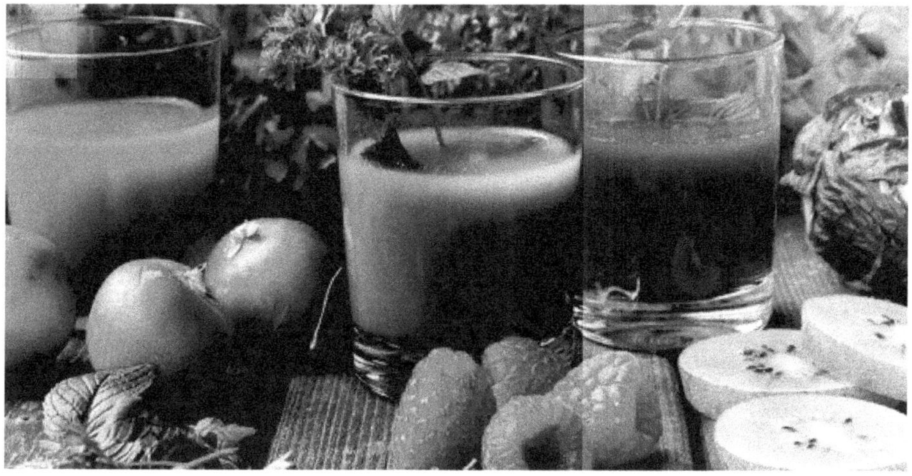

So ask yourself what is that sixth missing professional that we have so conveniently removed or ignored from our health "pac". Well of course it is the specialist from hence the medication came, the master herbalist. The Association of Master Herbalists, (AMH), recognizes herbal practice a form of Natural Healing which includes Herbal Medicine and a blend of Naturopathic techniques such as detoxification, nutrition, hydrotherapy, fasting and other ways to assist the patient back to health.

The master herbalist is a professional who is schooled, and has mastered the healing affects of herbs. Oddly enough we rarely think to consult an herbalist with the onset of an illness or disease. Ironically, this is should be the first cog in the wheel or the first of the "pac" that we consult before all the rest. Often, herbs, and naturopathic techniques can help the body to heal without the need for traditional medicines. I am not stating that an herbalist should take the place of a medical doctor or a chiropractor, physical therapist, nutritionist or psychologist. However I am stating that many times the herbalist can provide solutions to our heath problems that render these other professionals unnecessary. Therefore, making the absence of an herbalist in the health "pac" irrational, ludacris, and irresponsible.

Moringa Health corporate long-term vision, is to witness a day that they natural pathway to health is to seek out a local master herbalist as our "first choice" in health, and wellness. It is our hope that there will be a "herbalist board certification". Currently, in the United States, there is no certifying or licensing body in herbalism like there is for medical doctors, and thus there is no legally recognized certification or licensure for herbalists. Herbalists' right to practice, is protected by their right to free speech under the First Amendment of the United States Constitution.

Herbalists can educate clients on how to use healthful food, lifestyle practices, and herbs to support wellness and correct imbalance so the body can heal itself, but currently it is unlawful for herbalists to treat, cure, and prescribe as medical doctors can. We are seeing more, and more movement towards the recognition of herbalists. And it is encouraging as western medical doctors are slowly starting to embrace eastern ideologies, and herbal cures. Slowly more of their clients are moving away from first option pharmaceuticals, and are voicing a desire for a more holistic approach.

This pressure on the medical community is forcing some doctors to change their position on herbs and herbalism. However, the pharmaceutical lobby has a huge hold on doctors, and will continue to fight the will of the people and resist change. Fortunately the average person still retains the right to seek whatever medical modality and solution they deem fit.

Cost, often prohibit this, as insurance companies generally do not cover alternative health options. There are a few health insurance companies that are allowing alternative coverage. One called O'NA healthcare embraces all modalities, and preventative care. They do this buy being part of a tribal network and are able to credit deductibles for supplementation, and preventative health expenditures. (for more information contact Moringa Health)

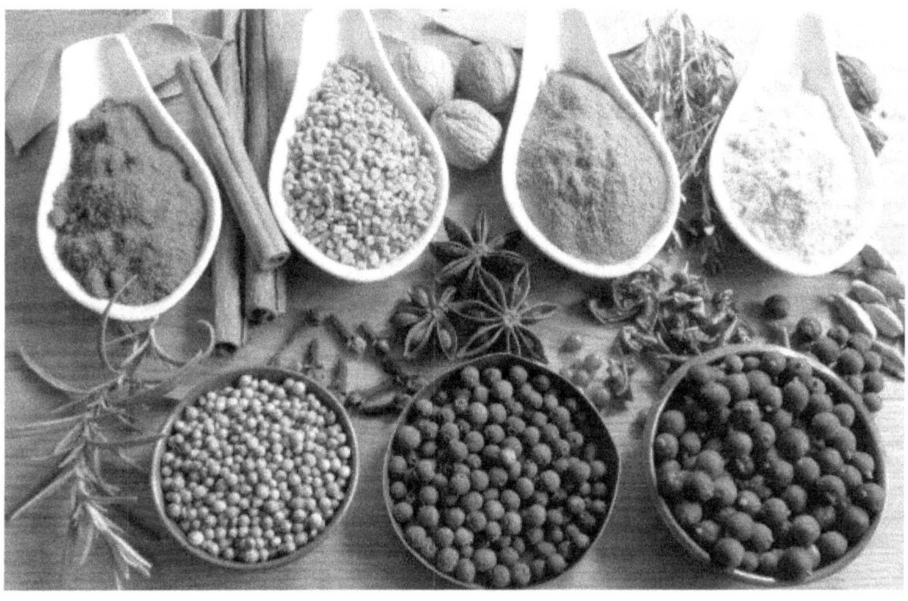

The American Herbalists Guild (AHG) is a professional organization that provides a peer-reviewed Registered Herbalist designation. While this does not have legal meaning like Board Certification for doctors, it does demonstrate that an herbalist has achieved a level of proficiency evaluated and recognized by professional herbalist peers, and some herbalists seek to achieve this designation. That being said, it is not a requirement for practice as an herbalist. Until there is board, and herbalism takes its rightful position next to medical physician, we recommend you seek out a Registered Herbalist prior to consultation.

Currently, when symptoms arise indicating an illness, we move first to a medical doctor. More often than not the medical doctor has little or no knowledge of herbalism, and will immediately move toward a pharmaceutical solution. Often not knowing if the prescribed drug will have a desired affect on the illness or not.

If the result is less than desirable the physician will simply prescribe another drug. The use of pharmacuticals as an initial solution, is often a calculated guess as the physician does not know the make up of our DNA, and how our individual bodies will react to the drug. In this way the medical professional is using our body as a "genie pig".

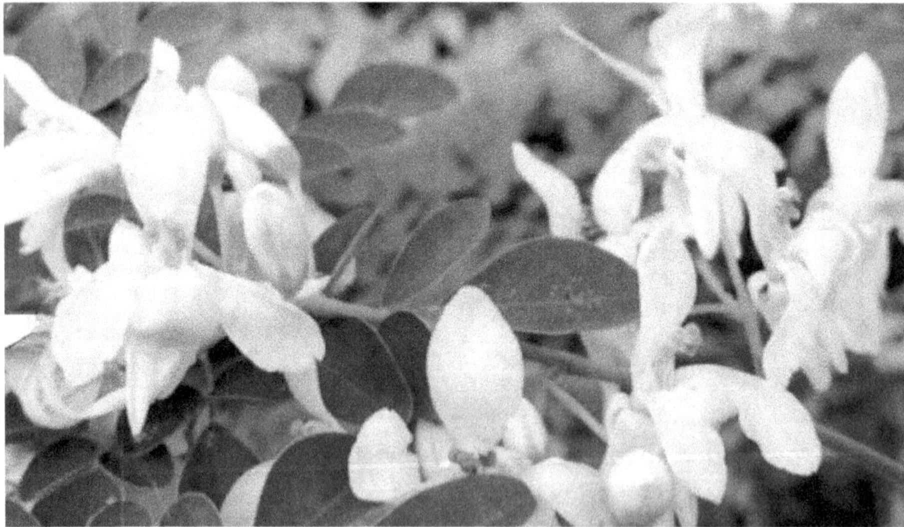

Ironically, these drugs deplete our bodies of much needed nutrients, and often create undesirable side affects. The true irony is that the herbalist, could have possibly provided an herb or combination of herbs that would provide the desired affect, while at the same time avoiding the negative side affects. Furthermore, if the herbalist was unsuccessful the result would not have put the patient through weeks of feeling worse, adding insult to injury.

On the contrary, the body would have acquired some form of benefit only without a reduction in the immune system or other negative side affects.

GODS TEMPLE

LIVING A HEALTHY LIFE

It is not my intent to aimlessly pontificate about what makes up a healthy life, but please allow me to take a moment to embellish. I am sure you know, that living a healthy life encompasses a spiritual, a mental, and a physical well-being. So the question arises, of these which is more important?

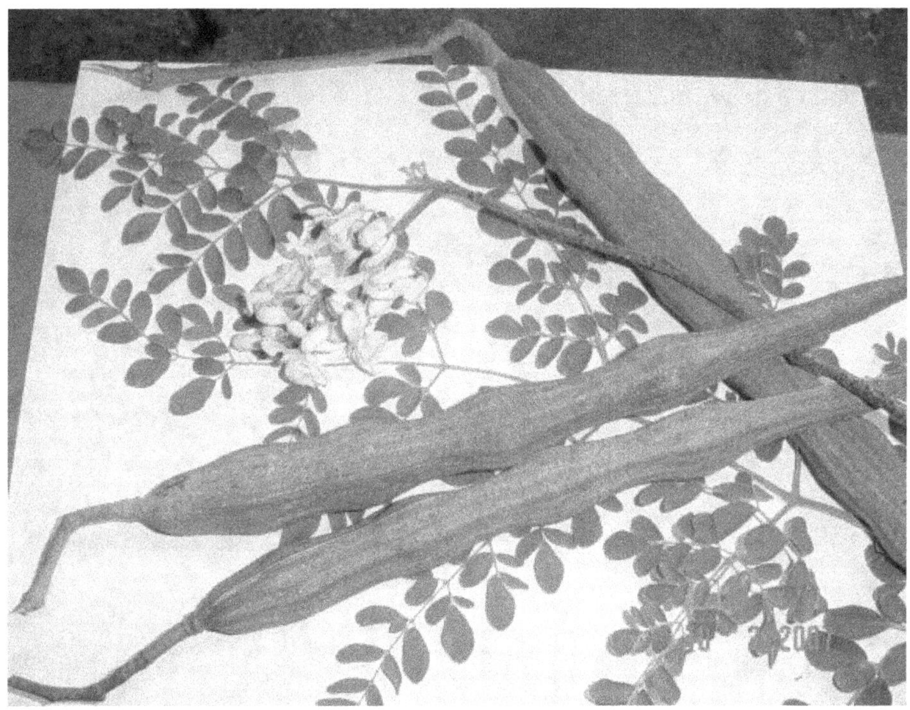

We could argue that our **spiritual health** is most important as it often dictates both our peace of mind, and our sense of purpose. How can one be truly healthy without having inner peace, and with a lack of an understanding of the lingering questions as to, why "I" am here. Other arguments could debate that our mental health is critical to our sense of consciousness, and our inter-action with reality. After all if you don't even know you exist, who you are, or have the facility to communicate, and have rela-tionships, how healthy could we be?

Finally, there is physical health. Certainly this has got to be the most important. After all how many times have you heard people say, "if you don't have your health you have nothing", or "if all I have is good health I would be happy". How healthy you are is of course super important. Your health dictates the quality of your life, and your energy level, and physical ability to enjoy it. One thing is for sure, physical health is integral to living a health life. No matter what your position here, I think we can all agree that spiritual health, mental health, and physical health are all instru-mental to how healthy we are.

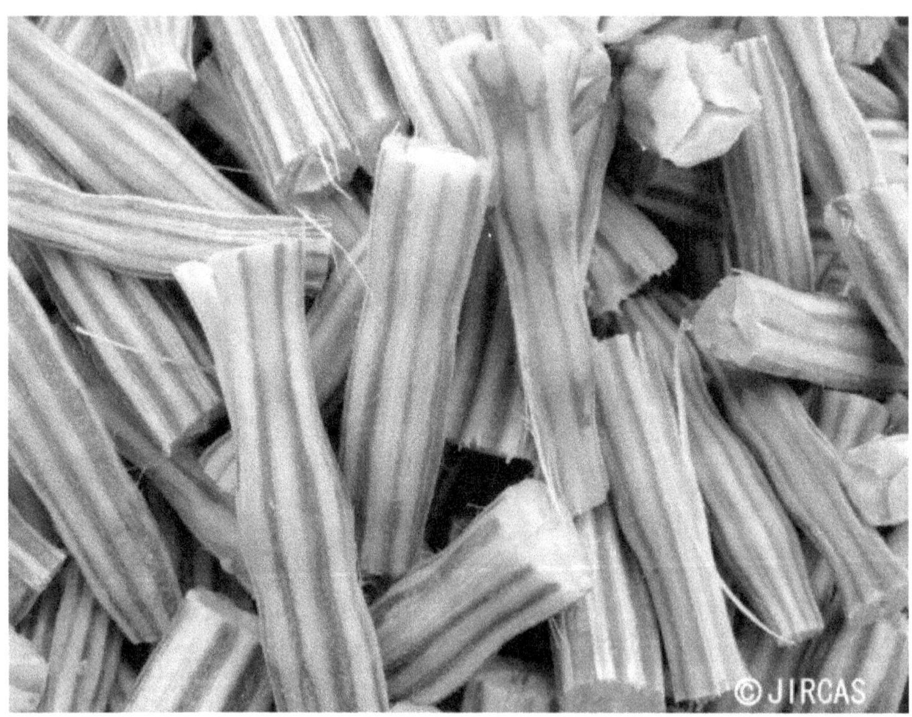

Through simple name association the "Miracle Tree"; could indicate that there is a spiritual element, and in its simplicity entice you to make moringa part of your daily regimen. Of course this is a bit of a reach, as name association is not true evidence of spiritual health. I would certainly concede to that notion. However, I implore you to research this miraculous tree, and after your do diligence I am sure you will come to the same conclusion that I have. That this tree is a true miracle, and gift from God himself.

Evidenced in that every part of the tree is edible and, every part of the tree can be used for some medicinal purpose. Numerous anecdotal studies have shown that this tree can treat more than 300 diseases, contains more than 90 nutrients and has 45 antioxidants.

Finally, Moringa leaf itself "leaves" (no pun intended), a feeling of well-being to its users. I am comfortable saying it is a spiritual felling of well-being and your "religious" use of this product is divinely ordained.

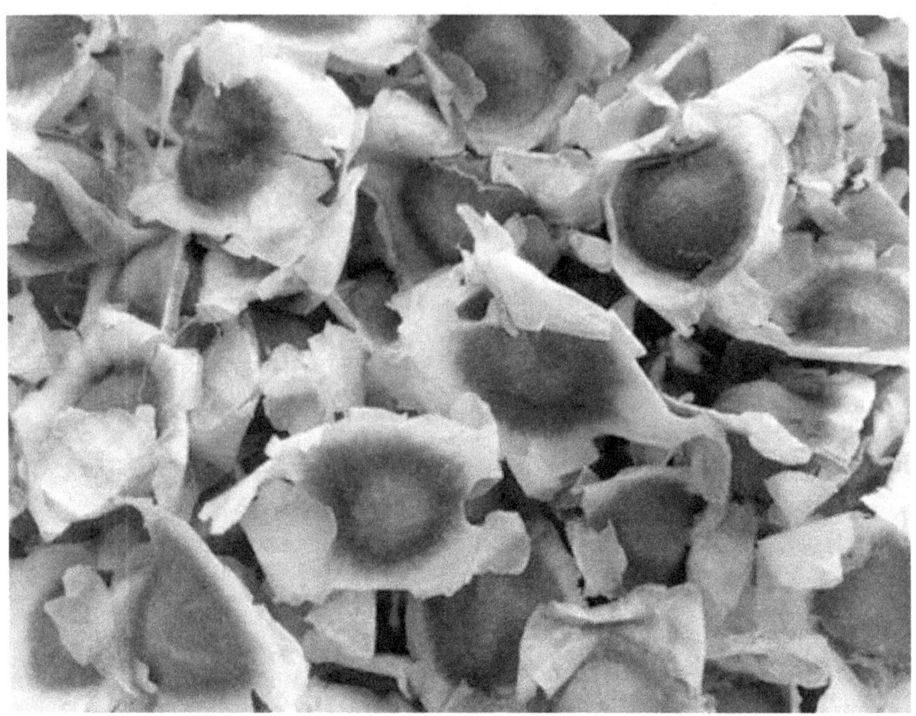

Our mental facility encompasses our ability to think, to reason, to communicate, to create, and to love. Mental illnesses are health conditions involving changes in thinking, emotion or behavior (or a combination of these).

<u>Mental illnesses</u> are associated with distress and/or problems functioning in social, work or family activities. I am by no means stating that moringa will cure mental health problems. However, I am stating that it will enhance your current mental health. The powerful concentration of nutrients in moringa will enhance your cognitive awareness, clear your mind, increase your blood flow, increase your mental energy, and improve your recovery in sleep. If the spiritual benefits were not enticing enough, I hope that your mental health and your mental capacity will incite you to action; so that you start using moringa daily, for you and your family.

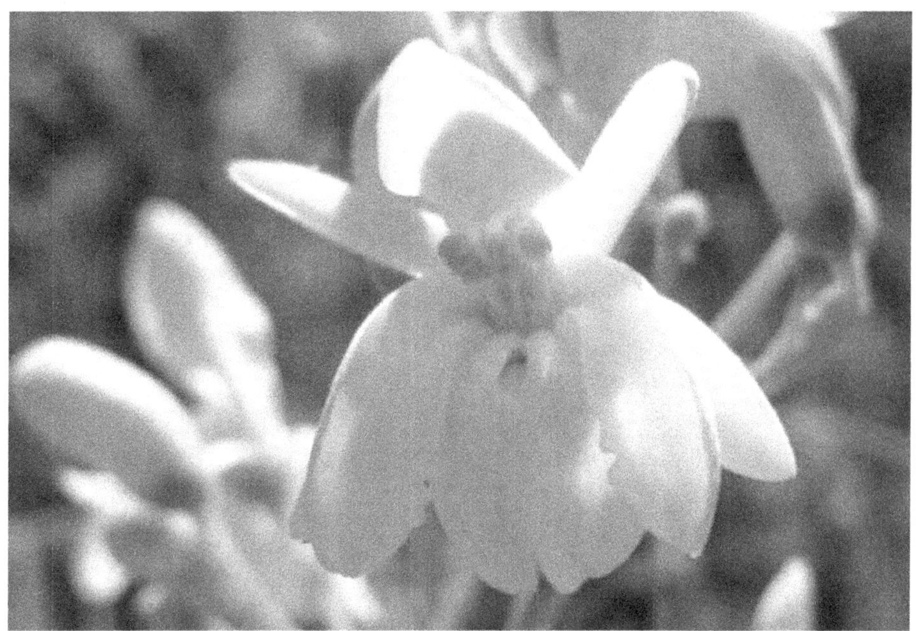

Moving one to action is the key focus of all motivation books, and speeches. Taking action is the catalyst to change and often moves us to positive result. Often change requires a physical action. In this case the ultimate goal of this book is to get you, and your family to take physical action. By ingesting both moringa capsules, and moringa based formulations created by the most reputable USA grown moringa product company,

Moringa Health.

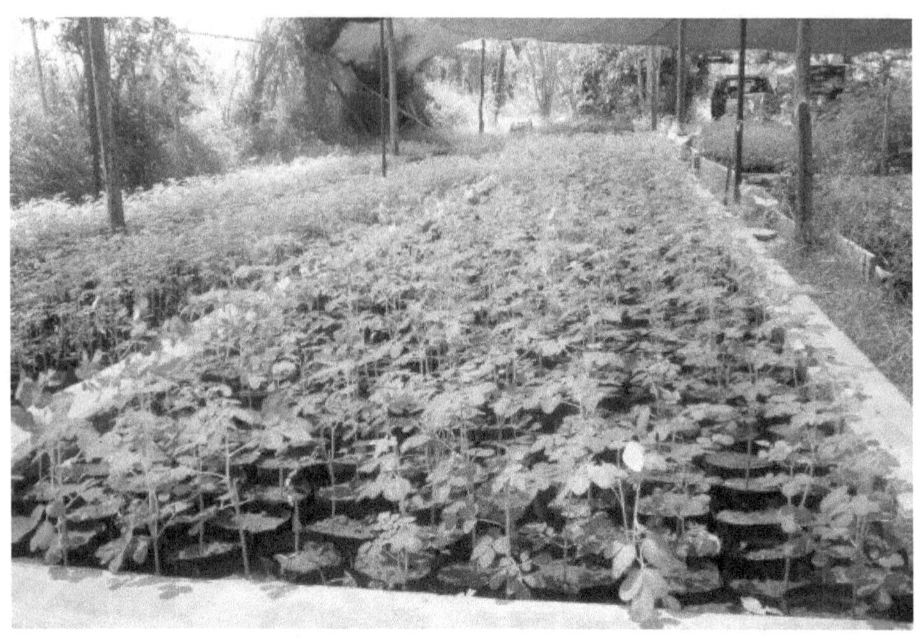

This leads us to the third pillar of health our physical health. Our physical beings encompass all that we are in the flesh. The saying 'you are what you eat", is often true and how we feel and function spiritually and mentally is directly tied to how we feel physically. Physical health is often associated with movement, and the act of physical fitness.

Our **physical fitness** determines how well we handle stress, how much energy we have, and how well we function mentally. Sleep, exercise, and physical intimacy all are determined by how we feel. Our body is dependent on proper nutrition to complete the full circle of our total physical health. So when you think about it the number one thing we can do to enhance our quality of life, and ultimately be health spiritually, mentally, and physically; is to get proper nutrition. What we eat, how much we eat, when we eat, and even who we eat with is essential to our over all well-being. So if you knew that there was something that you could eat, that could kick start your metabolism, cleans your internal organs, support your digestive system, improve you cognitive awareness, reduce the chance of disease, give you more energy, make you more productive, stimulate you libido, and enhance your felling of well-being; what would you do to get your hands on it?

Thank you for taking the time to read this:

I f you want to purchase any of our great products simply go to www.MoringaBenefits.org

May God bless you richly and abundantly.

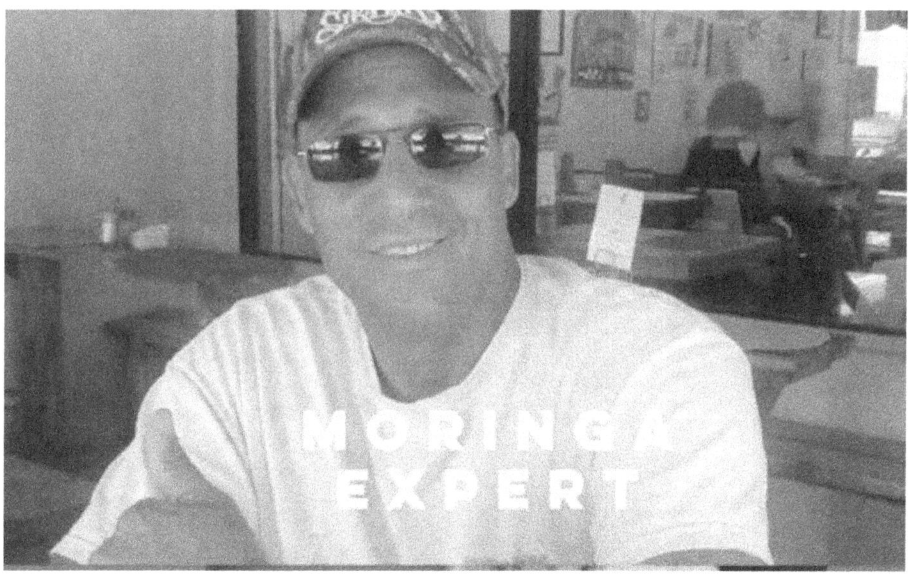

Douglas "Moringa" Mollo
Founder
Got Questions For Moringa Health?

Just Email Me : moringahealthrx@gmail.com

Message us here for any questions. Or to get a free sample of one of our amazing products.

https://fb.me/msg/douglas.mollo.56

Store: www.MoringaBenefits.org

Book Published and Edited by Brian Brown

Do Life Big Network www.dolifebigger.com/book